Praise for

The Anxiety Opportunity

To be anxious is to be human, for humans have indeed been anxious for as long as we have been on this earth. Moreover, each generation must address how it will respond to anxiety. Thanks be to God, Curtis Chang has not written a prescription *for* it; rather, he has opened for us a doorway *into* it—a doorway that leads to God, who is in all earnestness waiting for us in the very presence of our anxiety. Waiting to transform how we imagine it, which will lead to our becoming more deeply loved and beautifully transformed into the likeness of Jesus. For all of us who live with urgent anxiety, I invite you to allow what you hold in your hands to usher you through that doorway into comfort, confidence, and an opportunity to create the beauty and goodness that God longs for you to share with him.

CURT THOMPSON, MD, author of *The Deepest Place*,
The Soul of Desire, and *The Soul of Shame*

We are living in an age when anxiety is sweeping us further into a polarized, rage-filled world to escape the fears we refuse to name. Curtis Chang is a brilliant and winsome reader of the soul and body and what every honest human being suffers in anticipation of loss. His reframing of anxiety as an opportunity to know our own hearts and even more the kindness of Jesus will bring rest even in the fear-storms we all face. This tender, theologically vibrant, and psychologically wise gift is not merely for those who suffer anxiety; it's for every human being who longs to know more of what it means to taste joy.

DAN B. ALLENDER, PhD, professor of counseling psychology and
founding president, The Seattle School of Theology and Psychology

Anxiety is a widespread but not well understood condition. Curtis Chang, who has struggled with anxiety throughout his life, has written a book on anxiety that is sophisticated and sensitive, transparent and vulnerable, practical and faithful. *The Anxiety Opportunity* helps readers think about anxiety differently—constructively and biblically. Curtis has given us a gift—showing us how a problem can become an opportunity for spiritual growth. He has written a marvelous and necessary book.

PETER WEHNER, senior fellow, The Trinity Forum; contributing opinion writer, *New York Times*; contributing writer, *The Atlantic*

Anxiety anticipates loss. Loss is unavoidable. But in a hopeful and personal book, Curtis Chang argues that we are held even in our loss and anxiety by a God who loves us and who will make all things new. I was encouraged by Chang's description of prayer, grieving, and community as holding practices that can replace the avoidance habits that lock us into anxiety. This book is a practical guide that is also a witness to grace.

WARREN KINGHORN, MD, ThD, Duke University Medical Center and Duke Divinity School

The
ANXIETY
OPPORTUNITY

BOOKS BY CURTIS CHANG

THE ANXIETY OPPORTUNITY:
How Worry Is the Doorway to Your Best Self

ENGAGING UNBELIEF:
A Captivating Strategy from Augustine and Aquinas

The
ANXIETY
OPPORTUNITY

HOW WORRY IS THE DOORWAY
TO YOUR BEST SELF

CURTIS CHANG

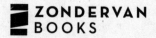

ZONDERVAN BOOKS

ZONDERVAN BOOKS

The Anxiety Opportunity
Copyright © 2023 by Curtis Chang

Requests for information should be addressed to:
Zondervan, *3900 Sparks Dr. SE, Grand Rapids, Michigan 49546*

Zondervan titles may be purchased in bulk for educational, business, fundraising, or sales promotional use. For information, please email SpecialMarkets@Zondervan.com.

ISBN 978-0-310-36731-4 (audio)

Library of Congress Cataloging-in-Publication Data

Names: Chang, Curtis, 1968- author.
Title: The anxiety opportunity : how worry is the doorway to your best self / Curtis Chang.
Description: Grand Rapids : Zondervan, 2023.
Identifiers: LCCN 2022051289 (print) | LCCN 2022051290 (ebook) | ISBN 9780310367284 (trade paperback) | ISBN 9780310367291 (ebook)
Subjects: LCSH: Anxiety—Religious aspects—Christianity. | Worry—Religious aspects—Christianity. | Spiritual formation. | BISAC: HEALTH & FITNESS / Mental Health | RELIGION / Christian Living / Personal Growth
Classification: LCC BV4908.5 .C395 2023 (print) | LCC BV4908.5 (ebook) | DDC 152.4/6—dc23/eng/20230217
LC record available at https://lccn.loc.gov/2022051289
LC ebook record available at https://lccn.loc.gov/2022051290

Cover design: Studio Gearbox
Cover photo: Marionn / Romashka2 / Ensuper / Shutterstock
Interior design: Denise Froehlich

Printed in the United States of America

23 24 25 26 27 LBC 5 4 3 2 1

To Jody, Faith, and Ellie

Contents

Preface

I'm worried.

    You'll read about more examples of my anxiety in this book, but here's one to kick things off. I'm worried that I will fail to include in these acknowledgments someone who deserves mentioning.

One of the ideas in the book is that every anxiety points to an outcome that is ultimately inevitable. That is certainly the case with this particular worry. Anxiety started affecting me as an eight-year-old and continues to be found in every aspect of my life today. If I tried to list every friend and thinker who has shaped my approach to this topic, I will certainly omit someone important.

So I shall instead restrict myself here to a narrower and more recent story—how those countless and nameless (by necessity) influences coalesced into this book.

This more specific origin story begins in the first weeks of the COVID pandemic of 2020. While I am a theologian and a former pastor, my primary vocation at that time was—and in many ways still is—in the broader secular world. I founded and run a consulting firm that serves secular nonprofits and government agencies. In that role, I lead a leadership development program that brings emerging nonprofit leaders together in monthly retreats. The first pandemic lockdown in our area was announced a few days before our March 2020 retreat and plunged everyone into unprecedented fear and uncertainty.

My colleague Kris Starr-Witort and I scrambled to shift the retreat format into Zoom. But it was obvious we also needed to scrap our previously planned retreat topic and address the anxious state of our leaders. With little time to prepare, I fashioned (with Kris's help) the new curriculum out of my own insights and experiences. The core content of the book took shape that day.

The tone of this book was also shaped by that origin story. From the start, I had to translate my insights—which were thoroughly permeated by biblical truths—for a secular audience. The gospel addresses the human condition, and there are few conditions more universal than anxiety. I hope this book will remain faithful to its origin and feel relevant to people from a wide range of spiritual backgrounds.

While seeking to remain accessible, this book does connect the universal experience of anxiety to a relationship with Jesus. My process of narrating this spiritual connection more explicitly took place in the context of The River Church Community in San Jose, California. Many years ago, I served as the lead pastor of this church—before my pastoral career was abruptly ended by a catastrophic episode of anxiety. You will read more about this episode in the book, but the fact that I remained as a lay member of this church (a rarity for ex-pastors and their former churches) testifies to the special nature of this community.

Brad Wong, the current pastor (he's the one who succeeded me in that role and also happens to be one of my closest friends) invited me to lead his staff team through the material. I partnered with my wife, Jody (more on her below), to develop and facilitate a staff retreat that integrated more explicitly Christian spiritual practices and truths.

After that retreat, Brad and other staff encouraged me to replicate the experience for the wider church community, since so many were struggling with worry during the first months of the COVID crisis. Since Jody and I could not personally lead dozens of live retreats, I realized that this anxiety material was converging with another effort of mine called Redeeming Babel. Before the pandemic, I had founded Redeeming Babel to develop video-based curriculum to equip Christians to engage fruitfully with the challenges and the opportunities of the secular world.

The Redeeming Babel team was indispensable in turning the retreat into The Anxiety Opportunity video course. I owe special thanks to Kris Carter (who helped me launch Redeeming Babel) and Josh Kidwell (who did the filming and postproduction work). Aryana Petrosky continues to lead promotional efforts and support the course (and now the book) in many critical ways. I'm also grateful for the expertise generously provided by our public relations consultants Heather Cirmo and Heather Douglass at Pinkston.

The final evolution from the video course to book was encouraged by Nancy French, the director of communications at Redeeming Babel. Since she herself is a *New York Times* bestselling author, I only agreed to undertake this project if she would serve as my initial editor. She was—and is—a joy to work with. Her skill, sensibilities, and enthusiasm have thoroughly influenced the book.

Nancy also helped me find my agent, Chris Park of DeFiore and Company. In turn, Chris did a fantastic job in guiding me to my publishing home at Zondervan. In my first exploratory meeting with Zondervan's publisher Webster Younce, I sensed an immediate fit. That sense was further confirmed when I started working with my assigned editor, Andy Rogers; his thoughtful input has made this book so much stronger. Thanks also to the wonderful Zondervan team of Katie Painter, Sarah Falter, Matt Bray, Paul Fisher, Denise Froehlich, Curt Diepenhorst, Paul Pastor, and Dirk Buursma who have supported this book with shared passion and their varied expertise.

I said I could not mention everyone who shaped my thinking about anxiety, but I must make a few exceptions. I have the privilege of being close friends with several extraordinary mental health professionals: Gilles Bekaert (MFT), Dr. Marsha Wadley (EdD), and Dr. John Q. Young (MD, PhD). Over the years they've not only shared key insights with me but have also cared for me directly during various personal crises in my life.

Finally, I come to the person in my life who has contributed the most to this book—my wife, Jody. At this point, my propensity for worry takes the form of the question, "How can I possibly describe how much she has meant?" As mentioned, she was my partner in the development of this content from early in the process. In every subsequent stage from retreat to course to book, she has read countless drafts, given invaluable feedback, and supplied needed encouragement. She's wise, candid, and caring. This book would not have happened without her, and it reflects the many ways we are truly "better together."

CHAPTER 1

A Surprising Opportunity

I was a latchkey kid.

If you didn't grow up in the 1970s, you may not be familiar with this phrase describing a child who comes home from school before parents return from work. Parents gave their kids a key with the expectation they could take care of themselves until dinner. I did just that starting at age eight—I walked home from my suburban Chicago school and let myself into our red brick house on Harvard Terrace.

At least that's what I was supposed to do. What I actually did was worry. My anxiety started when I unlocked the door. I had two older sisters, but my school let out before theirs. So I always entered the empty house alone with a sinking sensation in the pit of my stomach. I could never shake the scenario that someone could have broken into the house and would be lurking inside. How could I know that it hadn't occurred?

I waited by myself until one of my sisters came home. We had one of those old houses that made creaky sounds at odd moments. Occasionally, I heard what sounded like a step from the attic, and my heart started racing. I sometimes even rushed outside and sat in the front yard until a sister came home. When they asked me what I was doing outside, I shrugged. "I just wanted to play in the yard."

I felt better once my sisters were home. But as the afternoon approached evening, and we awaited the return of our parents, my anxiety would reignite. I worried that something bad would happen to my parents on their way back home.

I concocted a pretty clever plan to help me deal with these fears. My dad generally picked up my mom from the downtown bank where she worked until around 5:00 p.m., so every afternoon at 5:30, I called my mom's office.

"May I speak to Johanna Chang?"

"She's left for the day." My mom's coworker's voice was helpful and cheery.

"Oh, do you know what time she left?" I tried to make it sound casual, to hide the concern gurgling in my stomach. This was back in the day when bank workers would physically clock out on a machine, so her coworker would check the time on the machine and tell me when she had left.

Armed with her precise departure time, I calculated when my parents should arrive at home down to the minute. It was easy math. The commute averaged sixty-five minutes, and normally they arrived like clockwork. But if that anticipated arrival time passed, my anxiety would mount moment by moment until their white Buick LeSabre rolled into the driveway.

One day, a massive snowstorm hit Chicago, and the normal arrival deadline came and went. Then another hour and another.

This was before the cell phone era, so my parents couldn't alert me of the delay. I paced by the window, watching friends play in the snow. My parents were never going to arrive. Images of the three Chang children foraging for food filled my mind.

Who would we live with if they never showed up? My neighbors? I prayed we wouldn't have to end up with the crabby lady in her bathrobe across the street who smoked Marlboro Reds on her porch.

But my parents did finally pull into the driveway. They had survived for me to worry about them another day. And the day after that.

I never told my parents about this elaborate routine. In my eight-year-old brain, I sensed I shouldn't be calling Mom's coworkers and checking up on her. I sensed I shouldn't even be feeling this way.

One day, I called her office at 5:30 as usual, but—instead of a coworker—my mom answered the phone.

I panicked.

To cover myself, I pretended to be a bank customer. I don't remember exactly what I said. Since I was only in the second grade, my mind probably went to the bank commercials that aired during Cubs baseball broadcasts.

"So I'm just checking on what interest rates look like today," I might've said. "Maybe do a refi on the mortgage."

Mom played along—I'm sure she was trying to figure out what I was doing—and we talked for a few minutes. Finally, I ran out of things to say. "Well, uh, thank you, Mrs. Chang. I need to go now." But I still had a nagging question. "By the way, when are you leaving for home today?"

My scheme was blown.

She stormed into the house sixty-eight minutes later. Not that I was counting.

"So you thought it would be funny to fool your mom, did you?" She assumed I was pranking her and being disrespectful.

I looked at my shoes and nodded in silence.

She punished me for lying, and I accepted the punishment

without protest. I could not bring myself to explain to her what was going on inside. I never told her. Perhaps at some level, I didn't recognize the depth of the anxiety that was driving me. Or I didn't have the words to express it. Or perhaps, at a deeper level, I did recognize I was anxious but was too ashamed to admit it.

As I grew older, I developed much more sophisticated coping schemes. I evolved into what some psychologists call "high-functioning anxiety," which involves practices driven by anxiety that help you be successful in the world.

I became adept at staying on top of tasks, thinking several steps ahead, anticipating issues, coming up with fallback plans quickly. I excelled at school, got into Harvard, and graduated with honors. Only in retrospect have I realized how much my success was driven by this anxiety. I thought I was simply successful.

But like my "call the bank" ruse, coping schemes for anxiety run the risk of eventually getting blown.

Coping schemes for anxiety run the risk of eventually getting blown.

In my late thirties, I replaced the founding pastor of a large church in Silicon Valley and became senior pastor. I suddenly faced the pressure of preaching regularly and leading the church through a rocky season. Turns out, it is difficult to replace a founding pastor. Then the dot-com bust hit, the church hemorrhaged members, and we had to lay off staff.

None of my high-functioning anxiety practices could stem the sense of mounting failure. I felt I was in way over my head because I was.

For two weeks straight, I couldn't fall asleep. I may have had microsleep, where I went into sleep mode for a few minutes in the technical sense, but I don't remember falling truly asleep during that entire period.

I had panic attacks at inexplicable moments. For example,

my wife, Jody, and I took our two young daughters to a Halloween pumpkin patch—a pumpkin patch for toddlers, mind you; not one of those haunted houses for teens. Yet in the parking lot, I started to hyperventilate. The thought of entering the pumpkin patch was overwhelming. The world was closing in, and I was suffocating.

"Can you take the girls into the play area by yourself?" I muttered the words to Jody with a grimace and closed eyes.

"What's wrong with Daddy?" My daughters exchanged worried glances. I couldn't even find the breath or the words to answer. I remained in the car, gasping, alone . . . and ashamed.

Eventually, the anxiety slid over into depression, which can happen with severe and prolonged anxiety. My depression was so dark that it disabled me from doing even very basic tasks. I took a lengthy medical leave from my pastoral role, sowing confusion in the congregation. I could barely function as a parent. Jody shouldered the load for practically everything, from handling the girls' bedtime routines to shopping for groceries to paying the bills.

The experience was devastating. It ultimately ended my career as a church pastor. Could I ever work again at any job? If I couldn't even take my own children through a pumpkin patch, what in the world could I do for the rest of my life? The fear—and the shame—overwhelmed me.

I share all of this to say, *I know anxiety.* I know firsthand the suffering involved. While anxiety of any sort feels terrible, even functional anxiety doesn't feel good. In large doses, anxiety can cause immense damage, as it did in my life. Anxiety is not a good thing. And yet, there is more to the story.

Anxiety: A Short History

The American Psychological Association defines anxiety as "an emotion characterized by feelings of tension, worried thoughts, and physical changes like increased blood pressure." Anxious people may have "recurring intrusive thoughts or concerns. They may avoid certain situations out of worry. They may also have physical symptoms such as sweating, trembling, dizziness, or a rapid heartbeat."[1]

This condition has affected everyone since the beginning of time. In classical antiquity, Greek and Roman physicians and philosophers classified anxiety as a medical disorder. Ancient Epicurean and Stoic philosophers advised people on how to achieve victory over their anxieties.[2]

In subsequent eras, anxiety would be reported under different names. For example, Nitsuh Abebe reports that doctors in the nineteenth century described a nervous condition called "neurasthenia," thought to be caused by the accelerating pace of industrialization. Its symptoms included fatigue, worries, and irritability. Abebe quotes Andrea Tone, author of a book called *The Age of Anxiety*, as saying that this condition "was regarded . . . as the price Americans paid for their stunning success." The psychologist William James began calling it "Americanitis."[3]

In 1895, Freud wrote about "anxiety-neurosis," which occurred when fear attached itself to any idea. He wrote, "A woman who suffers from anxious expectation will imagine every time her husband coughs, when he has a cold, that he is going to have influenzal pneumonia, and will at once see his funeral in her mind's eye."[4]

In 1947, W. H. Auden captured the spirit of his time in his long poem titled "The Age of Anxiety," which won a Pulitzer Prize.[5]

In 1955, a muscle relaxer called Miltown became a popular anxiety antidote in Hollywood and New York, where martinis were served, garnished with Miltown pills. Lucille Ball, Tennessee Williams, and Norman Mailer bragged about consuming the new drug nicknamed "Executive Excedrin." Bob Hope dubbed it the "I don't care" pill. Tiffany & Co. sold jeweled pill cases so women could carry them in style.[6]

In the 1960s, Valium became the tranquilizer of choice, and anxiety—and its medicinal coping mechanisms—became a staple of songs. A 1966 Rolling Stones song called "Mother's Little Helper" dealt with the popularity of prescription tranquilizers among housewives. "Mother needs something today to calm her down," they sang. "And though she's not really ill, there's a little yellow pill."[7]

When Xanax became the stylish way to fight anxieties, musicians sang about that too. In 2004, U2 released a song called "Xanax and Wine." In 2007, Lil Wayne rapped, "I am a prisoner locked up behind Xanax bars."[8] In 2012, Whitney Houston reportedly died from Xanax (in a deadly cocktail of three sedatives that also included Ativan and Valium).[9] In 2013, Jason Isbell sang about his friend who took enough Klonopin—yet another medicine designed to help ease anxieties—to "kill a man twice his size."[10] Even more recently, Billie Eilish sang a song about Xanax abuse among her and her teen friends—a song titled "xanny"—in which she said that taking the pills caused a mental confusion that made them "too intoxicated to be scared."[11]

In recent years, all kinds of new terms emerged in the national discourse—terms such as racial anxiety, climate change anxiety, and election anxiety. As writer Matt Haig tweeted, it was difficult to tell "where your anxiety disorder ends and where actual news begins."[12] In the era of smartphones, *doomscrolling* entered the vocabulary to describe how we can get addicted to consuming information that makes us feel worried. We can't seem to stop ourselves from feeding our anxiety.

Anxiety has become the most common mental illness in the United States. In 2018, 63 percent of American college students reported overwhelming anxiety,[13] and COVID-19 made it worse. One study revealed depression globally rose 28 percent above pre-pandemic levels.[14] Some seek help through their churches, but "only 30 percent of pastors feel well-equipped to help congregants deal with matters of mental or emotional health."[15] Only 36.9 percent of those afflicted with anxiety seek assistance through medication or professionals, which means the vast majority are isolated and confused.[16] Many mental health experts believe we will be living with elevated levels of anxiety for years to come.[17]

•

I'm glad you're reading this book. We may indeed be in the midst of an "anxiety pandemic" in terms of increased intensity. But as our short history indicates, the condition has always afflicted humanity in some way.

Think for a moment. Was there ever a period in your life when you were free of anxiety? Has a year ever gone by in which you felt absolutely zero concern about the future of the world? Has a month ever passed by when you never felt even a stab of worry that perhaps you were failing or falling behind at something? Has a week ever passed without a moment of unease about what someone else may be thinking about you or whether someone is displeased about something you said or did?

All humans exist somewhere on the anxiety spectrum. On one end of the spectrum, some individuals live with so much anxiety that it feels like it's a part of who they are. Some may have been officially diagnosed with an anxiety disorder. On the other end, people balk at any description of themselves as "anxious," preferring to describe themselves as "occasionally stressed" or by some other label. Many people fall somewhere in between—people who may admit to a tendency to anxiety in certain situations or around certain topics, but not in or around other situations or topics.

Regardless of the intensity, regularity, or labeling of your anxiety, we've all suffered this condition. It is a universal human problem.

But here is the little-known truth about anxiety: it isn't only a *problem* we wish would go away; it is also an *opportunity* for spiritual growth. In fact, for a Christian, anxiety is one of the most powerful opportunities for transformation we'll ever encounter. My most transformative growth as a follower of Jesus has happened because of anxiety. This doesn't mean anxiety is good—that would be a ludicrous idea for anyone who has experienced anything similar to what I experienced at the pumpkin patch. Anxiety is not good, and even a book called *The Anxiety Opportunity* should not pretend that it is good or claim that God causes this condition for our good.

> Anxiety isn't only a *problem* we wish would go away; it is also an *opportunity* for spiritual growth.

But Jesus is our Redeemer, which means he can redeem something that is not good originally into something that benefits us ultimately. With Jesus, we can experience anxiety as an opportunity for transformation.

This truth is evident from my own life. I'm able to share this book with you now because Jesus is accomplishing in me his redemption of anxiety. I've seen it in the lives of countless followers of Jesus, and this opportunity is confirmed by Scripture itself.

It doesn't have to end in sleepless nights, ruined careers, or secret shame.

Anxiety can be used by God to transform your life with a blossoming of spiritual growth.

A Different Approach

Taking advantage of this opportunity requires us to think differently about the relationship between anxiety and spiritual growth. Broadly speaking, Christians have been taught to consider anxiety in one of two ways—either as an *obstacle* or as *irrelevant* to spiritual growth.

In the "anxiety as an obstacle" approach, you tend to imagine you are stuck on earth in your worries, while Jesus is in the heavens somewhere looking down reproachfully. Anxiety is viewed as a problem, as a flaw, perhaps even as a sin indicating you don't trust Jesus. It is evidence of a lack of faith. It's like me as a kid looking down at my shoes, feeling there was something wrong with me for being anxious.

The "anxiety as an obstacle" approach thus prescribes methods to get rid of anxiety as quickly as possible. The methods of elimination are spiritual in nature, such as "just having faith," "praying anxiety away," or "meditating on a particular Bible verse." Anxiety is then supposed to vanish. Once you push anxiety away, only then are you free to grow closer to Jesus.

In the "anxiety as irrelevant" approach, anxiety is treated as only a mental health condition to manage by "nonspiritual" methods. Anxiety and spiritual growth are separated. In many secular mental health approaches, spiritual growth is fine, but that's supposed to happen somewhere else, like at a church, a yoga studio, or on your own personal time—it is irrelevant to treating anxiety. The primary goal of mental health treatment is to lower anxiety. Common anxiety-lowering methods are therapy (especially what is known as cognitive behavioral therapy) and medication.

Let me be clear. The particular methods prescribed by both

"anxiety as obstacle" and "anxiety as irrelevant" all have value. Prayer, faith, and Scripture meditation are absolutely critical, and this book will cover various ways to engage in these practices when we are anxious. I also want to emphasize that we absolutely should treat anxiety as a legitimate health condition. I have benefited from both cognitive behavioral therapy with secular therapists and medication prescribed by doctors. I am all for lowering anxiety through these medical means.

But even some secular mental health leaders are starting to recognize that treating anxiety solely as a problem is counterproductive. Listen to Dr. Tracy Dennis-Tiwary, a leading researcher in the field:

> As a clinical psychologist and neuroscience researcher, I have devoted the past 20 years to understanding difficult emotions like anxiety, and I believe that we mental health professionals have made a terrible mistake. We've convinced people that anxiety is a dangerous affliction and that the solution is to eliminate it, as we do with other diseases. But feeling anxious isn't the problem. The problem is that we don't understand how to respond constructively to anxiety. That's why it's increasingly hard to know how to feel good.[18]

Both Christian and secular approaches miss "anxiety as opportunity"—the ways we can grow spiritually *through* anxiety. Anxiety is not an obstacle to spiritual maturity. It is not some moral flaw we must get rid of in order to grow toward Jesus. Anxiety is also not irrelevant—as if our mental health were disconnected from our spiritual health. Anxiety can be the very place where we meet Jesus. Through anxiety, we can actually become more like him.

The "Clobber Verse"

You've heard it.

The most commonly cited verse about anxiety is Philippians 4:6: "Do not be anxious about anything, but in every situation, by prayer and petition, with thanksgiving, present your requests to God." Among Christians, this is the verse most often wielded by the "anxiety as obstacle" approach.

Dr. Dan Allender, professor of counseling psychology at the Seattle School of Theology and Psychology, cautions the use of this verse in addressing anxiety. He says Philippians 4:6 can often be used by those who aren't experiencing anxiety as a means of "'clobbering' those who are anxious." Dr. Allender warns against "the idea of hearing Philippians 4 and assuming 'my anxiety goes away.'"[19]

I happen to like Philippians 4:6, but I also don't like how it is used as a "clobber verse" to make anxious people feel like they're doing something wrong or, even worse, that there is something wrong about them. As with most clobber verses, in this situation it is being used out of context.

To understand the verses in Philippians 4, you have to grasp the teachings of the previous chapter, which presents the theological core of the entire letter. Philippians 3 sets the overall context for Paul's words in 4:6 about anxiety and, in fact, establishes a key framework for how Christians should understand all aspects of their life.

The framework of Philippians 3 is that Christians live as "Now and Not Yet" people. This is sadly undertaught in Christian circles, which is why anxiety is so often misunderstood and why many clobber verses are misused.

What is a "Now and Not Yet" person? This person is summarized by Philippians 3:21, which declares that "our current lowly bodies are being transformed to the body of Christ's glory." The Now and Not Yet life is defined by the life goal of becoming like Jesus. This is the amazing promise of the gospel: God is at work to transform every bit of ourselves to conform to Jesus, the one who will give us his "glory." *Glory* is the biblical term describing the amazingly good way of life when we fully reflect God's intentions for us. Jesus obtained his glory because he fully reflected God's intentions in his life. Philippians 3:21 promises that as we become like Jesus, we will share in that same "glory."

However, the same verse assumes that this glorious destiny requires an understanding of spiritual growth that allows for the struggles of our current "lowly bodies." Note that *lowly* in Paul's usage here means "incomplete" (it does *not* mean "sinful"). He is emphasizing that the full completion of our transformation awaits the future, the Not Yet when Jesus returns (Philippians 3:10). In the Now, we will still struggle with experiences like the complex physical and neurological misfirings that were behind my hyperventilation in that parking lot. My current "lowly body" will still fall quite short of "glory."

Nevertheless, the Now and Not Yet are organically connected. This connection is missed entirely by the "anxiety as irrelevant" approach. My hyperventilation was not disconnected from my future glory; rather, in a mysterious way, it constituted the raw material of my transformation. This is what it means that our current lowly bodies are *being transformed* to the body of Christ's glory. Our Not Yet body of glory grows out of our Now body of struggle.

Paul isn't making up this Now and Not Yet dynamic. He gets it straight from Jesus. Jesus often used agricultural metaphors to convey this dynamic of spiritual growth. His favorite metaphor was to point to how a seed of some plant is growing in the present Now and still is on its way to becoming its fully completed self in the future Not Yet (see, for example, Matthew 13:3–8, 19–23; Mark 4:3–9, 14–32; Luke 8:4–8, 11–15; and more).

Because this is such a complex and crucial truth, Paul often adds to Jesus' agricultural metaphors for the Now and Not Yet. In Philippians 3, for example, Paul draws on the metaphor of a runner in the middle of a race, who is "straining toward what is ahead" (3:13) at the finish line. He switches to the metaphor of dual citizenship to capture the duality of the two time frames— living as citizens of the present earthly reality while awaiting the future arrival of a heavenly citizenship (3:20).

This overall "Now and Not Yet" framework is critical to understanding why Philippians 4:6 should not be wielded as a clobber verse that defines anxiety as a sin. Anxiety is an intrinsic and unavoidable feature of our Now and Not Yet incompleteness and should not be conflated

Incompleteness is not the same as sin.

with moral failure. Incompleteness is not the same as sin. We would be mistaken if we morally blamed an eight-year-old for being small or not knowing calculus . . . or for being racked with worry about their parents coming home.

In Paul's letters, he is not shy about calling out actions rightly labeled as sin and disobedience. But he's not using such moral categories in Philippians 3 and 4. For instance, the encouragement right before 4:6 is to "celebrate joyfully in the Lord, all the time" (4:4 NTE). But no one actually stays at this elevated spiritual state "all the time." We all regularly slip back down into more "lowly" moods.

Continual celebration is an aspirational description of the final transformation of our emotional self. While Christians are invited to taste more and more of those celebratory emotions here and now, I do not fall into sin when I stop celebrating joyfully in the Lord and, for example, lament the awful pitching of the Chicago Cubs. Paul describes periods when he is decidedly not in a celebratory mood but is instead struggling with deep despair (see 2 Corinthians 1:8, for example). He never labels those negative emotional experiences as sin.

Similarly, the encouragement right after Philippians 4:6 is to think only about holy, upright, virtuous things (4:8 NTE). Again, our minds will one day be transformed by the resurrection so we'll be able to accomplish this constant mental focus. In the meantime, we only sometimes experience periods of such a pure mindset, though we should aspire to have more of it. When our minds wander to, say, the latest celebrity gossip news, we have not committed wrong. Paul reveals how his own mind occasionally wanders to some fairly uncharitable (and crass) thoughts about his enemies. Galatians 5:12 includes some trash talking that would make a National Basketball Association player blush. Paul seems to accept these thoughts as part of his life in the Now.

In fact, those who wield Philippians 4:6 as a clobber verse to condemn anxiety as a sin neglect an important detail. Earlier in the letter, Paul describes his own anxiety for the Philippian church. Worry surrounded his decision to send his colleague Epaphroditus back to them. "This has made me all the more eager to send him, so that you'll see him again and be glad," he writes, adding, "and my own anxieties will be laid to rest" (Philippians 2:28 NTE). Having freely admitted his own anxiety—without a trace of self-condemnation—it would be bizarre for Paul to intend his words "do not be anxious" in Philippians 4:6 to be taken as an expectation that Christians would—or should—never feel anxious.

Therefore, in context, "do not be anxious" in Philippians 4:6 is not meant as condemnation; it is encouragement to experience anxiety within the larger "Now and Not Yet" dynamic of spiritual growth where our current lowly bodies are being transformed to the glory of Christ's body. Even as we aspire to more freedom from anxiety—an aspiration that will be met completely only in the Not Yet—we simultaneously should expect anxiety to always be part of our current life in the Now. We should no more expect Christians to be free of anxiety than we should expect Christians to be free of colds, mosquito bites, flat tires, sadness, or mental distraction. Paul brings up anxiety in Philippians 4:6 precisely because he expects it to be a persistent problem for his audience.

Those "lowly" experiences, far from being sins, are meant as signs. Your worries are like those people hired to dress up in a Statue of Liberty costume, twirling an arrow that points to a sale at a carpet store. These people can be annoying and distracting, but they are doing a job. They get our attention ("Look at me! Look at me!"), all the while redirecting you to the intended destination ("Go there! Go there!"). The Now and Not Yet person should be alert to ways that *current* and *lowly* experiences of anxiety serve as signs pointing to our future and complete transformation in Christ.

Or, to use one of Jesus' favorite metaphors, think of your worries as seeds. Anxiety anticipates some future payoff in the same way that tiny seeds of grain contain within them the anticipation of a future abundant harvest. Sometimes in our current lives, we get to sample an advance taste of this future payoff. In the Now, Christians can and do sometimes receive miraculous deliverance from anxiety. But any healing and deliverance are inevitably temporary on this side of the final resurrection. The healed person will still get sick and eventually die again; the person who was able to "pray away" one worry will inevitably struggle with another concern. Everyone must still await the final day when our healing and deliverance will be made permanent in Christ. Until then, there is always an incomplete, "Now and Not Yet" quality to our lives. Healing in the Now is always an anticipatory pointer to the final and permanent healing that only comes in the Not Yet.

The Bible expects Christians in the Now to get sick, suffer loss, and feel anxious. Those Now experiences are not evidence of moral sin; neither are they completely irrelevant to our spiritual destiny. Rather, these are expressions of our bodies still longing for the Not Yet. We were created for something better, and we are called to look forward to that future. Paul elsewhere describes how our bodies in fact join all of imperfect creation in "groaning" for our final redemption (Romans 8:22–23). My hyperventilation in the pumpkin patch parking lot was not me sinning; it was me groaning for transformation.

Therefore, this book does not promise that you can "pray your anxiety away" or give you some other technique to make your worries disappear. Anxiety most likely will be an ongoing— perhaps daily—issue for you as well. In fact, ironically, the more you accept this reality, the less anxious you will probably feel. But for a follower of Jesus, anxiety reduction is not the primary goal of life; our true goal is being transformed to the body of Christ's glory. This book will guide you to receive your anxiety as the seeds of transformation. You will learn to read your worries as signs calling for your attention and follow them to your ultimate destination: "Go there! Go there!"

CHAPTER 2

The Blueprint versus the Architect

Think back to a time when you encountered a new and unfamiliar setting. Do you remember the first time you had to navigate an airport and board a flight all by yourself? Have you ever had to check in at an unfamiliar hospital for a procedure? Or recall when you showed up on the first day of a new job?

Growing up in an immigrant family, we moved a number of times—and seemingly always at the wrong time in terms of school transition. There was a six-year stretch when I had to start at six new schools. Each school had a different way of lining up, a confusing layout, and, most of all, a sea of kids who all seemed to know each other—but not me.

Whatever example you've remembered, try to summon back those feelings of uncertainty and nervousness as you stood at the entrance. Now, suppose at that entrance, I gave you a choice between two options. The first option is to be greeted by a sign displaying a detailed blueprint of the place, with a precise "You are here" star and a clearly marked dotted path to direct you to your destination. The second option is to be greeted—to your great surprise—by a friend. You didn't know this, but it turned out your friend works here (or, in my example, goes to school here)! She warmly welcomes you with a hug and says, "Let me show you around!"

Which option do you want? It may seem obvious that the better one is the friend option. But when it comes to our life with God, it turns out that we tend to make the wrong choice.

Your life is filled with such entrances and this fundamental choice. Anxiety presents us with the opportunity to learn to choose better.

Meeting Jesus in Our Anxiety

Meeting Jesus is the starting point of all Christian spiritual growth. How then are we supposed to approach Jesus? Where in the varied situations of our life are we most likely to find him? This is where reading the Gospels is so helpful, for the stories of how people got closer to Jesus in the Bible are meant as models for how we can approach Jesus today.

I did my own study of how people approached Jesus in the gospel of Mark to see the larger truth about anxiety in Scripture.

I focused on the following groups of people who approached Jesus:

- people who approached Jesus (versus ones with whom Jesus took the initiative)
- people who approached Jesus in good faith (versus teachers of the law and Pharisees or other enemies)
- people who approached Jesus personally, either as individuals or small groups (versus "the crowds")

In the gospel of Mark, by my count, there are twenty-nine approaches to Jesus that met those conditions. Out of these twenty-nine, fifteen were marked by strong textual evidence of anxiety: (1) found in words explicitly describing anxiety (such as the word *fear*); (2) in Jesus' eventual response to the people in which he revealed what was really going on, such as when he says, "Peace . . ."; or (3) in actions strongly correlated with anxiety, such as a form of the verb *implore*, which conveys a state of emotional distress. These fifteen approaches to Jesus—more than half of the total—are clearly marked by anxiety.

Beyond these fifteen examples, an additional twelve approaches are marked by possible, if not definitive, evidence of anxiety. A good example is the story of the paralytic's friends in Mark 2 who opened a hole in a roof in order to get to Jesus. There is no explicit description of their anxiety, and Jesus comments on their "faith." But anxiety must have been present, since destroying someone's roof to get attention isn't the typical marker of people in a state of calm and peace! Classic anxiety behavior includes a narrowed thinking that disregards others, extreme behavior, adrenaline-driven physicality, and so forth.

Out of the twenty-nine total approaches, only two would be categorized as having no sign of anxiety. The first is the woman who, on the evening of Jesus' arrest, poured out the alabaster jar of nard in Mark 14. Her approach shows no evidence of anxiety. Jesus, remarking on her unique approach, says, "Wherever the gospel is preached throughout the world, what she has done will also be told, in memory of her" (14:9). She is an extreme outlier.

The second is Peter, who confidently declares, "I will never disown you" (Mark 14:31). Peter's expression of complete self-confidence is highly ironic and short-lived. A few sections later, when the cock crows in Mark 14:72, Peter is in a state of extreme anxiety.

Let this overall picture sink in for a moment. To repeat, the majority—more than half—of approaches to Jesus are undertaken by clearly anxious people. It is plausible to claim that almost all—twenty-seven out of twenty-nine—show some evidence of anxiety.

The evidence shows that people approach Jesus through a wide variety of anxieties. Out of the twenty-seven "strong or possible" cases of anxious approaches to Jesus, there are:

- eight cases of health anxiety
- seven cases of spiritual anxiety (especially around evil spirits)
- six cases of status anxiety (where a person is nervous about their standing or reputation before others)
- four cases of physical safety anxiety
- two cases of provision anxiety

The inclusion of this wide range of types of anxiety is deliberate. Mark and the other gospel writers are giving readers like you and me a variety of ways to locate ourselves in the overall story of people approaching Jesus.

The message is clear: people approach Jesus through their anxiety. Anxiety is not an obstacle and it is not irrelevant to getting closer to Jesus—it is the very entrance point for spiritual growth. Think again about the life situations that fill you with uncertainty and nervousness. It turns out that Jesus works there! He goes to school there! And there he welcomes us with a hug and says, "Let me show you around."

A Spiritual Tour of Anxiety

When we do meet Jesus in our anxiety, if we are at all attentive, he will show us the true nature of our condition. The medical profession provides various definitions of anxiety in tomes like the Diagnostic and Statistical Manual (DSM). These guides focus on the numerous behavioral and physical symptoms of the condition (like rumination or sleeplessness). But Jesus takes us deeper than just the symptoms; he diagnoses the underlying spiritual cause.

The best example of Jesus serving as the tour guide of our anxiety is found in the Sermon on the Mount. In Matthew 6:25–34 (ESV), Jesus says this to his followers:

> Therefore I tell you, do not be anxious about your life, what you will eat or what you will drink, nor about your body, what you will put on. Is not life more than food, and the body more than clothing? Look at the birds of the air: they neither sow nor reap nor gather into barns, and yet your heavenly Father feeds them. Are you not of more value than they? And which of you by being anxious can add a single hour to his span of life? And why are you anxious about clothing? Consider the lilies of the field, how they grow: they neither toil nor spin, yet I tell you, even Solomon in all his glory was not arrayed like one of these. But if God so clothes the grass of the field, which today is alive and tomorrow is thrown into the oven, will he not much more clothe you, O you of little faith? Therefore do not be anxious, saying, 'What shall we eat?' or 'What shall we drink?' or 'What shall we wear?' For the Gentiles seek after all these things, and your heavenly Father knows that you need them all. But seek first the kingdom of God and his righteousness, and all these things will be added to you.
>
> Therefore do not be anxious about tomorrow, for tomorrow will be anxious for itself. Sufficient for the day is its own trouble.

The spiritual essence of anxiety is summarized in the first verse of this passage: "Therefore I tell you, do not be anxious about your life, what you will eat or what you will drink, nor about your body, what you will put on" (Matthew 6:25 ESV). In the subsistence economy of Jesus' day, people lived with the possibility they could lose essentials like food, drink, and clothes. In our abundance economy, of course, we fear losing other things. Some of the things are bodily essentials, such as health, but our fear of loss encompasses more abstract things as well, such as status, a comfortable retirement, and a sense of belonging.

Anxiety is the fear of loss. Regardless of the nature of objects we fear losing, the spiritual essence of anxiety is our very human worry that we may lose something we value. Take a moment to think about a current worry that's bothering you. It could be something from your job, your family, your finances, the wider world, or some other realm. Try to be very specific in identifying the actual concern. Do you have it in mind? Now ask yourself, *What is it that I fear losing?* You can go back to the range of anxieties that Jesus welcomed in the gospel of Mark to diagnose more precisely your anxiety. Is it the fear of losing your health, some spiritual status, reputation, safety, financial provision, or something else? Try to name specifically the loss that you fear.

The fear of loss is the spiritual essence of anxiety. But there's one more key element—the timing of this feared loss. Notice how often Jesus emphasizes the *future* dimension of the feared loss—what you *will* eat, *will* drink, and *will* wear. If the importance of the future dimension of anxiety wasn't clear enough, he concludes his teaching by underlining it: "Therefore do not be anxious about *tomorrow*, for tomorrow will be anxious for itself. Sufficient for the day is its own trouble" (Matthew 6:34 ESV, emphasis added).

The fear of loss is the spiritual essence of anxiety.

Anxiety is about tomorrow, the future. Anxiety tries to make us fear something that could happen later. It is not about something happening right now.

Consider again the specific worry you just identified. Ask yourself, *To which time frame is this anxiety taking me? Is it the past, the present, or the future?*

Jesus would say every one of your anxieties abducts you from the present and carries you into some imagined future scenario. Even if the anxiety was triggered by a past event—for example, a disagreement with a supervisor last week—anxiety harasses you by projecting you into the future with an imagined scenario like, *What if my supervisor gives me a bad review next quarter?*

In my breakdown as a senior pastor, it may have seemed like I was concerned about the decline in church membership happening in the present. But in reality, my anxiety was all about the future: *What would it feel like to fail as a pastor? Would staff resent me for having to lay them off? And oh, what if I lose my own job?* And so on and so on . . . ever more into the future.

Think of anxiety as a kind of blueprint, the technical drawings used by architects and designers. When first drawn, the blueprint depicts a future scenario that does not yet exist in concrete reality; it is imaginary, only existing for now on the blueprint itself. The anxiety blueprint is a distinctive kind of blueprint because whereas all architectural blueprints depict a future scenario of gain—a new home or building that will be built—the anxiety blueprint is a future scenario of loss.

This anxiety blueprint is not fixed on a paper, of course; it is being generated by our minds. And because what is being drawn is a scenario of something that doesn't exist yet, there is no current reality to constrain what our minds can draw up. Anxiety can constantly revise its drawings. In periods of life when the future feels especially uncertain and unconstrained, anxiety can roam ever further into the future and devise one new scary scenario after another. The more we allow anxiety to draw and redraw such blueprints of loss, the crazier these pictures get, such that we can end up staring at the equivalent of a bizarre haunted house.

If I could have slowed my racing thoughts in the pumpkin patch parking lot and traced them calmly as an outside observer, I would have mapped a similar flight into the future that sounded something like this:

> *The pumpkin patch will have a maze to navigate. What if I can't do it? Will my daughters realize how messed up I am? What if they lose respect for me? What if I'm still like this when they grow up? Will I even be allowed to walk them down the aisle when they get married? Wait, marriage . . . what if my wife gets tired of my pathetic condition? She's not going to be able to tolerate all of this for much longer. She's going to leave at some point. O God, I am going to die alone. I'm going to be one of those corpses discovered weeks later by a landlord knocking on a door to collect the late rent!*

This mental flight from a pumpkin patch to my lonely death-bed may sound crazy, as if I had become detached from current reality. But that's the point. Anxiety pulled me from current reality. It's like I was staring so intently at a crazy blueprint of a haunted house that I became absorbed by it and started to mentally walk into it. The blueprint came to life in my mind. Its imaginary future of loss became my current reality—which is why my body responded as if I were actually losing my daughters, my wife, and even my life, and I started hyperventilating.

The Blueprint versus the Architect

So if the spiritual essence of anxiety is that it is a blueprint of a feared loss in the future, what is the spiritual answer?

One answer that many Christians instinctively want from God is this—a safer and better blueprint. We want the sign that assures us, "You are here" and a detailed pathway for our future. If anxiety scares us with its future scenarios of feared loss, then we naturally assume we'll find relief by gaining from God alternative future scenarios secured against loss. In other words, many of us are tempted to think we will feel less worried by trading out anxiety's blueprint for God's blueprint.

There is a grain of truth to this instinct. God does seek to transform our vision of the future; getting a new picture of the Not Yet is part of becoming the "Now and Not Yet" people described in chapter 1. But this transformation requires a process of spiritual growth. And the growth begins by distinguishing our desire for the blueprint from our desire for the Person behind the blueprint.

This is where we are invited to approach anxiety as an opportunity for *spiritual growth* and not just grab for immediate relief of psychological discomfort. If we desire spiritual growth, we have to realize that when we want a blueprint, we want a *what*—something essentially impersonal. The blueprint we want from God is one that promises we won't lose valued *things*—money, comfortable homes, reputation, health, and more. Even when our desired blueprint focuses on securing the ongoing presence of people in our lives (such as our spouse or our children), keep in mind that the blueprint itself is not the same as the personal reality of those people. The blueprint is a drawing that depicts those people; it is not those people in reality. Moreover, the blueprint is a drawing about the imaginary future, not the flesh-and-blood humans you hold and hug right now in the present.

When Jesus teaches about anxiety in Matthew 6, he realizes his listeners are fixated on getting the blueprint of our future as it pertains to things—*what* you will eat, *what* you will drink, *what* you will wear (verse 25). Notice what he does. He seeks to shift his listeners to the *who*. He redirects them to the present reality and character of their Father God. He summarizes this shift in verse 32: "For the Gentiles seek after *all these things*, and *your heavenly Father* knows that you need them all" (ESV, emphasis added).

Making this shift from desiring the *what* to desiring the *who* of your heavenly Father is a critical step of spiritual growth for any Christian. For our lifetime, we are not actually promised by Jesus many specifics about the *what*. The crowd listening to him is worried about what they will eat, but Jesus doesn't give them the Father's course-by-course description of their future meal plan. They are anxious about what they will drink, but he doesn't reveal their future wine inventory in their future wine cellar. They are nervous about what they will wear, but Jesus doesn't catalog their future wardrobe. Instead, Jesus reminds them they have a Father who cares for them, sees them, and knows them. There is an important difference between a heavenly Father and a heavenly supply chain.

This difference between the *what* and the *who* is the difference between a blueprint and an architect. A blueprint depicts a specific set of things that will be delivered in the future. An architect is the person behind those things. As Hebrews 11:10 declares, God himself is the Architect, the person who is the "designer and builder" of all things (ESV). Do we desire the blueprint? Or do we desire the Architect?

Anxiety is an opportunity for any Christian to grow from just wanting the blueprint to wanting the Architect. Many of us may have started our Christian life thinking that this new way of life was a blueprint for avoiding loss. That's okay. Jesus can work with that starting point, just as he worked with the crowds to whom he gave the Sermon on the Mount. But we can't stay stuck there. If you're not sure what spiritual growth means at this point in your life as a follower of Jesus, your anxiety serves as a great diagnostic. What you are seeking as an answer to your anxiety will reveal a great deal.

If the only satisfying response to our worries is the *what*— some scenario that promises we won't lose certain things in the future—then that means we really are still relating to God mostly with a view to getting a favorable blueprint from him. It's like we want to skip the process of first developing a close relationship with the architect; in our anxiety, we burst into the architect's office at the first meeting and demand that he turn over a blueprint immediately to assuage our fears. That is not spiritual growth. We need to become people who actually deep down want to get to know the Architect, the *Who* of God. This is true Christian spiritual growth.

Do we want this growth? This is Jesus' implicit question in Matthew 6. He's saying to his audience, "I know you want to make sure you have all these *whats*. I'm offering you the *Who*, the Great Architect, the one who designed and created you and knows you inside and out." This doesn't mean we don't ever ask the Architect for things—we will, of course, ask our heavenly Father for what we need. But a heavenly Father is so much better than a supply of things. In terms of spiritual growth, the question is what do we ultimately desire?

We need to become people who actually deep down want to get to know the Architect.

If we remain fixated on the *what*, the blueprint, we will gradually lose the *Who* of God. We will lose our access to the personal presence of God not because he will reject us or abandon us. He won't do that. But we will lose the personal presence of God because from our end, we will increasingly treat God as an impersonal mechanism. We will relate to our Father God the way we might relate to a computer printer that generates blueprints for the future. In facing anxiety, we will want the secret code, the right sequence of buttons to punch so that the printer will spit out the desired blueprint. Indeed, so much of the "pray anxiety away" teaching in the church can sound like instructions on how to punch the right buttons to get God to deliver the scenario we want.

We were made for something more. Or more accurately, we were made for Someone more. Anxiety is our opportunity to diagnose the true nature of our desires. And it is the opportunity to learn to choose better.

CHAPTER 3

The Hijack

When I was eleven years old, I watched a movie called *Raid on Entebbe*. The movie depicts the real story of the 1976 hijacking of an Air France jet airliner by terrorists. The hijackers landed the plane in the Ugandan airport of Entebbe, where they were welcomed by the country's dictator, Idi Amin. In response, the Israeli special forces developed and executed a daring rescue plan. The plan had several clever twists, including landing a plane containing the replica of Amin's limousine with a soldier dressed to resemble the dictator. This twist gave the rescuers the opportunity to penetrate the airport grounds, surprise the hijackers, and free the hostages.

The movie entranced me (notwithstanding the ludicrous casting of Charles Bronson to play an Israeli general). For weeks afterward, I replayed the movie in my head and fantasized about participating in the rescue plan. Lying on my living room couch, I wielded my Louisville Slugger baseball bat, which progressed in my imagination from an airplane throttle guiding our heroes into Entebbe into a reconnaissance telescope to peer outside the disguised limousine and then into a machine gun that killed the evil hijackers.

Many of us are currently engaged in a battle against hijacking. The hijackers are not of flesh and blood, but of the mind. This battle occurs not in childhood fantasies but in our real-life struggle with worries.

I've been emphasizing that anxiety is an opportunity and not *just* a problem. This is true. But it is also true that anxiety does present significant problems for us that require an immediate response. The most pressing threat posed by anxiety is how it hijacks our minds.

We need a rescue plan. This book provides you with one that works. We start this plan with a twist that confounds the hijacker.

Getting Present

Recall how Jesus gave us a tour of the spiritual nature of anxiety in the Sermon on the Mount. He explained how anxiety abducts us from the present and commandeers us into its future scenarios of loss. The time frame is critical. The future is the terrain where anxiety exercises its power over us.

When anxiety hijacks our mind into the future, we can be tempted to think we must fight on the terrain of the hijacker's choosing. We believe we can only combat anxiety by staying in the future. This is why we want God to give us an alternative blueprint of the future. Or we will work on devising our own scenarios, calculating probabilities, and devising potential actions.

"Cognitive behavioral therapy" is a mainstay of secular mental health because it trains people to do this in a highly structured way. And spiritually, as we'll explain later in the book, taking full advantage of the Anxiety Opportunity means letting God reshape our vision of the future in a profound way.

However, I have found that it is very difficult to reconfigure our imagination of the future—either through secular or spiritual means—when our minds are still in the tight grip of the hijacker. When we are in the throes of anxiety, such mental calculations easily get abducted into more worrying. We first need a twist in the rescue plan.

The first step in the plan is to *get present*. Leaving the future deprives the hijacker of its hold over us. We refuse to fight anxiety head-on in the future but instead walk away from that terrain altogether. Modern psychological research and therapy methods have validated this insight: *You cannot feel anxious when you are fully present.* When you read accounts of elite pilots, special forces operators, firefighters, and other highly trained individuals who face harrowing, life-threatening crises, they often describe a moment when they focus entirely on the task at hand. They refuse to be hijacked into the future and instead get entirely present.

You cannot feel anxious when you are fully present.

The power of getting present was dramatically shown on January 15, 2009, when Captain Chesley "Sully" Sullenberger and copilot Jeff Skiles accomplished one of the most miraculous emergency landings in history.

At 3:24 p.m., their flight was cleared for takeoff from LaGuardia Airport in New York City. Somewhere between 2,900 and 3,000 feet, the plane hit a flock of geese.

"Mayday! Mayday! Mayday! This is Cactus [1549]. Hit birds. We've lost thrust in both engines. We're turning back toward LaGuardia," Sullenberger radioed to LaGuardia. They advised him to return to the airport, but he was unable to make it. He attempted to target another airport, but he was plummeting to earth. "We may end up in the Hudson," he radioed. Seventeen seconds later, he delivered an unthinkable message: "We're gonna be in the Hudson."

The aircraft swooped over the George Washington Bridge, missing it by less than a thousand feet, before he landed the plane successfully in the Hudson River.

When later asked about this "miracle on the Hudson," Captain Sullenberger said he was able to pull off this amazing crash landing by focusing on the now:

> I never had any extraneous thoughts in those few seconds that we had. I didn't allow myself to and I didn't have any inclination to. I never thought about my family. I never thought about anything other than controlling the flight path and solving each problem in turn until, finally, we had solved them all. . . .
>
> I think . . . the training and the experience . . . develops in you an ability to summon up from somewhere within this ability to create a sense of calm, a professional calm.[1]

Elite personnel like Captain Sullenberger receive highly specialized training in how to get fully present. In Matthew 6, Jesus gives his audience a training method that is universally accessible. Here Jesus teaches his followers to leave the imaginary future, the time frame that makes them worried about what they will eat or drink or wear. If Jesus were speaking to a middle-aged crowd today, perhaps he might say, "For now, stop calculating the worrisome trajectory of your retirement account and the financial moves you may need to make in the next ten years." Instead, he wants us to get present: "Therefore do not be anxious about tomorrow, for tomorrow will be anxious for itself" (v. 34 ESV). Leave tomorrow—the future. Get back to today—the present. All of the specific encouragements Jesus provides in the Sermon on the Mount are invitations to his listeners to stop imagining fearful scenarios and be present to God in the here and now.

Jesus especially encourages people to learn how to get present by paying close attention to nature. He's telling them, "Look right now at the birds and the lilies around you." Everyone can access the natural world God created. Getting present to nature reverses the hijack from the shadowy future because nature is about the Now. It's the bee zooming around your picnic table, the squirrel munching on an acorn, and the grass growing taller than it was last week.

Nature organically leads us to get present to the Architect of all creation. Paying attention to creation reminds us that our present reality is filled with the Creator's loving care. Nature is filled with signs that God is constantly providing for his entire creation. Even if you live in an urban environment, you can walk outside right now and observe in nature a multitude of signs that God is constantly providing for us—from the very air that fills our lungs with life-giving oxygen to the sun that warms our skin. This is a powerful rebuttal to anxiety's bullying threats, which are usually about things being taken away from us.

The present reality of God's creation—not the shadowy, imaginary future—is the playground the Father designed for his children. The present reality is where our Father wants to take us.

Note that Jesus is talking about getting mentally present *to* nature, not just physically getting *in* nature. Sometimes when I get anxious, I vaguely remember that nature is helpful, so I put on my shoes and go outside for a walk. All too often, I use nature as a background scenery for anxiety. I'm walking outside, but I'm still allowing myself to be hijacked into the future. I'm still rehearsing all those shadowy scenarios—but I'm just doing it outside now.

Jesus encourages his followers to get present *to* nature. He tells us in Matthew 6:26, "Look at the birds of the air"—not in a distracted fashion as background scenery for our internal anxiety—but with intent. Looking intentionally means perceiving the true lesson seen in the life of the birds. They are small, fragile creatures sustained right now by the Father. Jesus tells us in verse 28 to "consider [really pay attention to] the lilies of the field" (ESV). Don't use them as background scenery for your anxious thoughts. Stop, observe, smell, and absorb their glory, their stunning beauty that reflects the Creator's care.

Try this now. Set a timer for sixty seconds, and for this duration, look out your window and really be present to what you see. Notice the shifting shape of the clouds, the particular hue of the sky, the fluttering shapes of the leaves, or whatever is present in your corner of creation. Notice as many details as you can.

After you've done this, consider how much anxiety you experienced during those sixty seconds. If you actually got present to nature like this, you should have experienced a minute of freedom from anxiety. If you can get present to nature, even for a few moments, you will not feel anxious. At least for a few moments. You cannot be anxious when you are fully present to God's creation. We were made to have this response. A large body of research shows that human beings seem to be hardwired at an unconscious level to feel greater calm in nature.[2] When Christians combine this unconscious wiring with a conscious appreciation of the Creator himself, they are armed with a powerful reminder of God's presence in the Now.

The more you do this in your life, the more you will free yourself from anxiety's hijack to the future. And the more you will open yourself to the loving, reassuring presence of the Father—just as Jesus promised.

The Mindful Breath

In addition to getting present to nature, a second powerful and Jesus-centered way to get present is the *mindful breath*.

The practice of mindful breathing has become popular in the broader culture. You may have practiced mindful breathing at a work meeting, in a yoga class, or in any number of other settings. Some Christians are uneasy about mindful breathing out of fear it originated from spiritually problematic sources. But this practice has a profound biblical basis.

John 20 shows how mindful breathing can be traced directly to Jesus. At this point in the story, Jesus has been crucified, resurrected, and has even appeared to the disciples. However, the disciples are in a state of intense anxiety. John 20:19 states that they are cowering behind locked doors "for fear of the Jewish leaders." They are being bullied by imaginary scenarios of the future where they are arrested and perhaps even crucified like their leader.

Jesus appears suddenly among them as they huddle together in their anxious state. Once again, we see that anxiety is the meeting ground for Jesus. Pay close attention to what happens next in John 20:21–22 (emphasis is mine): "Again Jesus said, 'Peace be with you! As the Father has sent me, I am sending you.' And with that *he breathed on them* and said, 'Receive the Holy Spirit.'" Jesus is being "mindful" in his actions here. His action of "breathing" is deliberate, not some throwaway, random detail.

The mindful breathing of Jesus physically embodies what is happening spiritually: Jesus is giving them the Holy Spirit. Jesus is about to leave the disciples physically and will not return until some unknown time in the future resurrection. But he won't leave them—or us—alone.

Jesus will return to us physically at some point in the future.

But in the meantime, we are not latchkey kids. The Holy Spirit is how Jesus will continue to be present to the disciples. Likewise, Jesus is still present to us in the Now through the Holy Spirit as we await the Not Yet of his physical return. John 20 shows that this gift of the Holy Spirit is tied up with the physical act of mindful breathing.

The mindfulness of Jesus' breathing becomes even more apparent when you realize Jesus is tapping into a long tradition in the Scriptures where God's sustaining, constant presence is embodied in breath. This tradition goes all the way back to Genesis 1:2 where the "Spirit of God" hovering over creation is *Ruach Elohim. Ruach* is "breath" in Hebrew. *Ruach Elohim* is literally the "breath of God."[3]

Jesus' emphasis on breathing embodies our "Now and Not Yet" life with God. Breathing embodies how the Holy Spirit is with us for every present moment of "the Now." Our breath will be with us for every present moment of our life. As you read this, you are breathing. As sure and real as your breath is now, so is the presence of Jesus with you through the breath of the Holy Spirit. Through the Holy Spirit—the *Ruach Elohim,* the breath of God—Jesus is present with us. Right now. The more you practice Jesus-centered mindful breathing, the more you can stay in the Now and resist anxiety's hijack to its imaginary future.

Breathing also embodies how God will be with us in his "Not Yet" reality. Our future transformed bodies will also be filled with breath supplied by God. This is the inevitable conclusion drawn from the promise that our current lowly bodies are being transformed to be like Christ's glorious body (Philippians 3:21). The resurrected body of Christ was breathing in and out. Therefore so will our resurrected body. We will physically breathe with our eternal lungs. And we will not be gasping alone. We will be breathing peacefully and mindfully with Jesus.

Anxiety may seek to bully us with all sorts of imagined scenarios of our future—most of which will never take place. Far more assured is the reality of our coming life in and with Christ. As we practice mindful breathing, we remind ourselves of our assured "Not Yet" future. We replace anxiety's threats about the imaginary future with God's promises about the real future found in our resurrected Lord.

Mindful breathing is how we physically enact the "Now and Not Yet" presence of Jesus. This is why Jesus-centered mindful breathing is a powerful defense against anxiety. Rich spiritual truths undergird the practice, yet the action is itself amazingly simple and accessible. We don't need to think about all of these truths while we're practicing mindful breathing. The physical act itself embodies the truth.

Getting Present to the Who

Practices like getting present to nature and mindful breathing are highly effective ways to immediately lower our anxiety levels. But we're missing the full opportunity if we only practice them solely for symptomatic relief.

The deepest benefit of getting present in these ways is growing our relationship with God. No relationship can be built in an imaginary future. When we are encouraged to "get present" with a spouse or a child, we can't do that if we're only relating to them about what they should do for us in the future. We can only grow a personal relationship in the present—by being present to that person in the here and now.

For example, suppose I'm anxious about my financial future. This means anxiety is hijacking me to a scary future where a tanking stock market is eroding my IRA. Suppose I meet you at a party for the first time. We talk for a few minutes and then I say, "Okay, got it, your name is Eric, you're married to Martha, you have two kids and whatever, but look, where do you think tech stocks are headed? You don't know? Well, what about good real estate investments? Nothing? How about crypto?"

Imagine I do that not just to you but to every person I meet at the party? How superficial, how thin, how false! Word would quickly get around that I'm not actually interested in developing a relationship with anyone.

Yet that's the way many of us are tempted to relate to God in our anxiety. We stay in the future because we want to avoid loss in the future more than we want to embrace a Friend in the present. Spiritual growth is about a relationship with a loving God, and no intimate relationship grows in the imaginary future. Relationships only grow in the present—when we get present to the other. It is true with other humans. It is true with God.

God does care about our future, and he does want to give us a future. As we cultivate our relationship with God through Jesus, our very understanding of our destiny will be transformed (which will in turn transform our experience of anxiety, as we'll see in later chapters). But it is a profound mistake to fast-forward past this cultivation—which only happens in the Now—in a rush to obtain from God a reassuring blueprint of our Not Yet. When we skip past the Now, we will likely envision—and demand from God—an incorrect Not Yet that is more a projection of our fears than the true intention of God. God's future for us grows out of a present relationship with Jesus. We have to start in the Now.

In the throes of anxiety's hijack, you will be motivated to engage in the practices of getting present to obtain symptomatic relief. By all means, build these practices on this initial motivation to just feel better. But as you do so, look for the ultimate payoff, our highest good. One sign of spiritual growth is increasingly experiencing Jesus himself as your ultimate desire and treating symptomatic relief as bonus add-ons. To paraphrase Jesus in his teaching on anxiety in the Sermon on the Mount, when you seek first him as the highest object of your desires, "all these things will be given to you" (Matthew 6:33).

As you allow the Anxiety Opportunity to take you to the Who, you can end up in a reality deeper than just feelings of symptomatic relief. Indeed, you may end up beyond even the realm of subjective feelings and thoughts entirely. When I recovered from the period of intense anxiety and depression that ended my pastoral career, I experienced what the Christian spiritual tradition calls a "dark night of the soul."[4] The "dark night" refers to what many Christians throughout the centuries have experienced—a prolonged period where God seems absent.

I suppose it wasn't surprising I would undergo this feeling of divine absence: I had for so long experienced God in the context of my ministry, and I no longer had a ministry. Related to being a minister, I also engaged with God primarily through words and well-formed concepts. For most of my life, my prayer life was highly verbal in form (my most "effective" form of prayer was usually journaling), and I felt God responding when a theological idea came to me.

Words and concepts about God were inaccessible during the "dark night of the soul." For me, the attempt to formulate words in prayer suddenly felt like an exercise in futility, even almost ludicrous. Well-ordered theological ideas did not flow back to me, only silence.

Anxiety and depression do not always lead to the "dark night of the soul." But my conversations with other Christians indicate that for many, this is a pattern that occurs. Perhaps it is enough to recognize anxiety and depression are forms of suffering, and those who suffer deeply rarely emerge unchanged. The "dark night of the soul" announces the passing of the old and portends the arrival of the new.

My spiritual life changed. Out of the futility and silence, I gravitated to an ancient practice known as contemplative prayer. Contemplative prayer eschews verbiage and thoughts and embraces silence. It practices a presence of God deeper than words about God. It is akin to how sometimes I am most present to another human being in silence. For example, I can lie in bed at night next to my wife, not exchanging a word, and still feel close to her. God can be powerfully present to us in silence as well.

One anchoring practice of contemplative prayer is mindful breathing. In contemplative prayer, breathing is not about combatting anxiety per se; it is a way to quiet mental distraction and draw the person back to the presence of God. Because I was already practicing mindful breathing in my recovery from the symptoms of anxiety, I found it natural to transfer the activity into this new context of prayer. My anxiety became the practice grounds for this new spirituality.

Contemplative prayer has become a mainstay of my life with God. The practice has become a portal into a deeper experience and exploration of God's presence. This presence goes deeper than the realm of subjective feeling. In contemplative prayer, you may feel very little. Your thoughts may be random and fleeting. But you trust that God is nevertheless present at a deeper level, present objectively beyond your feelings, your thoughts, your subjective experiences. The absence of these things gives way to the presence of Another. The anchor of one's spiritual life increasingly sinks past the shifting sands of oneself and instead hooks into the objective bedrock of all reality, God himself.

Perhaps I would have eventually found my way here without anxiety and depression. But God redeemed my suffering in profound ways to bring me to this place. As you follow the Anxiety Opportunity, you may or may not end up in the specific practices of contemplative prayer (although I hope you'll be willing to be taken there if God invites you). But you will be changed. Suffering changes everyone. Even though this book recasts anxiety from solely being a problem to make go away, it doesn't promise to eliminate the painful aspects of anxiety. Anxiety is still a form of suffering. But it is a suffering that can lead to deep, profound change. We follow a crucified Lord who suffered greatly and emerged from his suffering utterly transfigured. And in this Now and Not Yet life, our "lowly bodies" are drawn into this redemptive dynamic. Our anxiety participates in the presence of the one who suffered, and the one who changed.

CHAPTER 4

The Shame of Anxiety

B all four!"
It was the fourth straight batter I walked after being summoned from the bullpen. Four of four. My first outing as a Little League pitcher was already a disaster. The infielders behind me groaned in exasperation. I glanced sideways into the stands to see parents of my teammates shaking their heads, and my own parents—immigrants who didn't fully comprehend American baseball—looking confused. My mind raced forward to what everyone would think of me if I continued to fail like this.

My heart raced, my breath constricted, and my muscles tightened. I wanted to flee from the mound, but the coach didn't budge. I was trapped.

My next pitch sailed five feet over the head of the catcher, clanging against the backstop. The pitch after that skipped well short of the plate, kicking up a cloud of dust.

I needed an out. Not a strikeout—no chance. I needed a psychological way out.

I made a big display of adjusting my cap, readjusting it, and readjusting it again. Surely, people would recognize the real problem was the incorrect angle of the brim of my cap that failed to shield my eyes from the sun. No? I held my glove over my forehead in a dramatic attempt to gain more shade. I strained my neck and squinted my eyes. Wasn't it obvious? Blinding solar rays were aimed directly at the eyes of the defenseless pitcher! Of course, my pitches were going astray. It wasn't anxiety—no, I was confronting an exploding supernova.

I walked that batter. And the next. Between each pitch, my exaggerated behavior resembled more and more what it would be like if Count Dracula had been summoned from his crypt to pitch in a day game.

I have no idea how I eventually secured three outs. The umpire probably started calling any pitch landing somewhere in the zip code of home plate as a strike. As I walked off the mound, I shrugged my shoulders the way I imagined a stoic soldier would as he departed a battleground filled with insurmountable odds.

I made it as far as the sidelines before I burst into tears.

Deflecting Attention

People struggling with anxiety naturally look for such outs. The adult versions are more sophisticated, but they are similar in nature. We are tempted to deflect attention to some problem "out there."

To be clear, real-life anxiety is often intensified by external factors that should be addressed. When we experience financial anxiety, we need to pay attention to the credit card statement and make all necessary spending adjustments. When we experience performance anxiety before a presentation, we should review the audience list, the setting, the material, and our notes.

However, we need to recognize anxiety as something inside

us and not just focus on solving external problems to make anxiety disappear. Indeed, we must recognize false and dangerous narratives that shift blame outward for our anxiety.

When I was trying out different therapists as part of my recovery from my catastrophic breakdown as a senior pastor, I had to narrate my problem with each candidate. With each one, I always began the narrative by describing those two weeks of total sleeplessness. In my initial retellings, I pointed to insomnia as the cause. But in reality, something like that almost never happens out of the blue. Anxiety must build over time to get to the point of collapse. The key is to recognize anxiety while it is still building within us.

Recognizing anxiety can be challenging. In the months preceding the collapse, I didn't identify my anxiety because I kept narrating what was happening to me as some problem out there—outside of me.

For instance, sleep disturbance is one of the most common signs of building anxiety. In the months

The key is to recognize anxiety while it is still building within us.

before my period of complete insomnia, I awakened way too early and was unable to fall back asleep.

During that buildup, I told myself the sleep problem was caused by a heavy workload and lack of time. My body, I told myself, was adjusting by waking early so I could get things done. Notice the narrative push "out there"—my workload was the problem, not the anxiety inside me.

When I couldn't get back to sleep, I'd ruminate about the conflicts with other pastors on my team. We were considering layoffs because of budget challenges, and another pastor had a different take on the issue. After one debate with him in a staff meeting, I awakened at three in the morning, replaying the debate in my head. I couldn't fall back asleep.

So I got up and composed a five-page email message explaining my position and critiquing his. Needless to say, he was taken aback when he read my late-night diatribe in the morning. He gently pushed back. *Why did you send me this long email in the middle of the night?* In retrospect, he was trying to get me to recognize that something was wrong inside me. But I didn't see it. I composed another email message, explaining that I needed to frame the problem correctly if I was to lead the team. Since the team was taking too long, I had to move things forward. Again, I was deflecting attention to all these problems "out there"—not recognizing the anxiety within me. I could not allow others or even myself to recognize my inner state. Left unrecognized, the anxiety kept building within me until I broke apart.

Why did I keep deflecting attention from my own internal anxiety?

The same reason my eight-year-old self could not admit to my mom what was going on inside me. The same reason my Little-Leaguer self kept pointing to the sun. A senior pastor is not supposed to be gripped by anxiety. A senior pastor is supposed to trust in God. A senior pastor is not supposed to fear failure at his first church or a slashed budget that can't pay the senior pastor, forcing him into homelessness! Such fears aren't supposed to keep a faithful, God-trusting senior pastor up at night, right?

In other words, I felt ashamed about my anxiety.

Shame is one of the most aversive feelings that humans can experience. Anxiety feels bad enough; adding shame on top of it makes the combination almost unbearable. So when we get anxious, we will be highly drawn to some narrative that deflects our internal shame into external blame. It was the sun; it was the workload; it was my super-slow staff team—anything but the brew of uncomfortable realities within me.

This shame-driven deflection is dangerous because it distracts us from recognizing the true nature of our problem and the true remedy. On a purely medical level, I likely could have avoided the catastrophic nature of my eventual collapse had I admitted my anxiety and sought psychiatric treatment (including medication) when

Deflection is dangerous because it misdirects us from the ultimate remedy.

my symptoms were still building. Instead, I wasted months doing things like writing self-justifying emails at three in the morning.

On a spiritual level, deflection is especially dangerous because it misdirects us away from the ultimate remedy. For Christians, the only lasting answer to our shame is found in Jesus' profound embrace of us, a welcome that encompasses our anxious self. We will explore how this works in our next chapter on acceptance, but the key insight for now is that we will miss Jesus' solution if we follow some narrative that pushes everything out toward external blame. Such a narrative is like a faulty sign pointing us away from Jesus because his acceptance of us takes place inside us—it doesn't happen "out there."

As a sidenote, we see the danger of this deflection impulse in the prevalence of conspiracy theories. The psychological factors driving large numbers of people to adopt false and irrational conspiracy theories are complex, but research has demonstrated a strong correlation with anxiety.[1] It seems that people who feel worried about losing economic or social status—and perhaps experience a sense of shame around that loss—are especially drawn to false narratives that blame some "other" group. Such people can get so thoroughly attached to these conspiracy theories that they essentially fuse their very identity with them. Friends and family members who try to reason with or fact-check these adherents usually make little headway because such arguments stay in the world "out there" and aren't addressing the underlying emotional drivers of anxiety and shame.

On both social and individual levels, we all need to recognize the anxiety that exists "in here" and start there. We see this response pattern in Jesus himself.

Jesus Recognizes Anxiety

In the gospel of Mark, an interesting dynamic emerges. When the person approaching Jesus narrates their problem as an external problem happening "out there," Jesus often refocuses their attention to their internal state. Jesus will deal with the external problem eventually; he's not ignoring it. But often, he first wants the person to recognize their own anxiety as the starting point.

Take a moment to read about one such example from Mark 5:21–42:

When Jesus had again crossed over by boat to the other side of the lake, a large crowd gathered around him while he was by the lake. Then one of the synagogue leaders, named Jairus, came, and when he saw Jesus, he fell at his feet. He pleaded earnestly with him, "My little daughter is dying. Please come and put your hands on her so that she will be healed and live." So Jesus went with him.

A large crowd followed and pressed around him. And a woman was there who had been subject to bleeding for twelve years. She had suffered a great deal under the care of many doctors and had spent all she had, yet instead of getting better she grew worse. When she heard about Jesus, she came up behind him in the crowd and touched his cloak, because she thought, "If I just touch his clothes, I will be healed."

Immediately her bleeding stopped and she felt in her body that she was freed from suffering.

At once Jesus realized that power had gone out from him. He turned around in the crowd and asked, "Who touched my clothes?"

"You see the people crowding against you," his disciples answered, "and yet you can ask, 'Who touched me?'"

But Jesus kept looking around to see who had done it. Then the woman, knowing what had happened to her, came and fell at his feet and, trembling with fear, told him the whole truth. He said to her, "Daughter, your faith has healed you. Go in peace and be freed from your suffering."

While Jesus was still speaking, some people came from the house of Jairus, the synagogue leader. "Your daughter is dead," they said. "Why bother the teacher anymore?"

Overhearing what they said, Jesus told him, "Don't be afraid; just believe."

He did not let anyone follow him except Peter, James and John the brother of James. When they came to the home of the synagogue leader, Jesus saw a commotion, with people crying and wailing loudly. He went in and said to them, "Why all this commotion and wailing? The child is not dead but asleep." But they laughed at him.

After he put them all out, he took the child's father and mother and the disciples who were with him, and went in where the child was. He took her by the hand and said to her, "*Talitha koum!*" (which means "Little girl, I say to you, get up!"). Immediately the girl stood up and began to walk around (she was twelve years old). At this they were completely astonished.

When Jairus first approached Jesus, he narrated his problem

as one that was "out there"—the health condition of his daughter back home. Natural and understandable. If I were Jairus, that's exactly how I would narrate my problem and my request. The problem is my daughter's illness, which is happening back there at my house, and my request is for Jesus to fix that situation.

Jesus accepts this man's initial approach and travels with him back to his home, the supposed location of the problem. On the way, they are interrupted by the woman with the flow of blood, a condition that automatically marked her for shame. The woman starts telling Jesus her whole story. She has been sick for twelve years, has tried many doctors, and is discouraged because nothing worked—and so on and so on.

As this woman's narrative of worries and shame drags on, you can imagine Jairus glancing at the position of the sun (since he didn't have a watch) and tapping his sandal-clad foot. *My daughter back at the house, my daughter back at the house, my daughter back at the house. That's the real problem, and this is taking too long.*

Some messengers arrive with bad news: Jesus is too late, Jairus's daughter is dead. Jairus's attention naturally goes even more to "out there" back at the house. I imagine he launches into questions about what happened there. "Are you sure? When did she die? Who is with her now?"

If Jairus believes the messengers' news, perhaps his mind switches to a "high-functioning anxiety" mode to deal with other external problems: "How am I going to comfort my wife? What kind of burial arrangements are we going to make? What will I say at the funeral?"

Notice Jesus' response. He interrupts Jairus's train of thoughts and redirects his attention. To where? To his internal state. "Don't be afraid," he says. Jesus directs Jairus to what is happening inside him. Jesus wants Jairus to recognize his anxiety.

This response is especially striking. Jesus could have said, "Jairus, I'm raising your daughter from the dead even as we speak. We don't even have to finish this journey." Jesus responded that way in another miracle with a centurion in Luke 7. But with Jairus, he doesn't even explicitly promise a specific external outcome. He doesn't say a word about how he will deal with Jairus's external problem. He directs attention solely to his internal state of anxiety.

Jesus cared about the dead daughter. Jesus cared about Jairus, whose pain is real and his situation heartbreaking. Jesus understands why it preoccupies Jairus, and he will eventually deal with her death with his resurrection power.

But first he wants to deal with the anxiety inside Jairus, which means Jairus must recognize what's going on inside him. The journey must go there.

Notice what this means. Jairus does not know exactly what Jesus is going to do to solve his problem. He has to walk all the way home with Jesus while dealing with his anxiety.

Try to imagine what that journey was like for Jairus because it represents our own anxiety journey. In our own life, all sorts of external problems will trigger our anxiety. And we will naturally want to focus our attention on finding solutions for those problems. We may even ask Jesus to fix those problems. In fact, trying to get Jesus to fix those external problems will absorb an enormous part of our spiritual energy.

Jesus understands our problems. And he will ultimately respond. He has a plan for those problems. The plan may or may not achieve the kind of solution we are seeking. Most of the time, Jesus doesn't tell us ahead of time, just as he didn't tell Jairus.

Before the plan is fully revealed, however, Jesus may first direct our attention to our own internal anxiety. He wants us to recognize what is going on inside us. Why? Because spiritual growth happens within us, not out there. From the soil of our inner anxiety, we grow closer to Jesus.

Back to the journey home. I envision Jairus and Jesus walking side by side. Jesus had essentially said, "Let's start with your state of fear, Jairus." In my imagination, Jesus now raises one of his eyebrows, tilts his head slightly, and smiles kindly. All of it signals, *Shall we talk about that?* The invitation hangs in the air.

How will Jairus respond? Will he keep focusing on an endless string of potential external problems? Or will he accept Jesus' invitation? Will he recognize his own anxiety and make his inner reality the topic of conversation with Jesus?

Mark doesn't let us in on how willing Jairus was to talk to Jesus on their journey. He leaves it open-ended. I think it is because we are supposed to insert ourselves into the journey.

Are *we* willing to recognize our own anxiety as we walk with Jesus? Are you?

CHAPTER 5

The Name of Anxiety

Both of my daughters experienced various challenges during their adolescent years. They sometimes struggled in peer relationships, in their enjoyment of school, and in their sense of purpose. In other words, they were contemporary American teens.

Fast-forward to today, and both are thriving, focused, and highly mature young adults. But back in high school, all of that lay in the unknown future, which meant that as a parent, I was vulnerable to potential scenarios born out of anxiety. Every problem seemed unprecedented and ominous. As a parent, my anxiety—which had been mostly manageable since my cata-strophic breakdown years earlier—reignited.

My anxiety manifested in all sorts of "out there" impulses, as I initially tried to resolve all of their social, academic, and existential problems. Surprise! Turns out, modern American par-ents can't fix everything for their daughters any more than Jairus could for his.

I began to ruminate. Rumination happens "in here," specif-ically in our minds. Rumination is the psychological term for a mental captivity to unpleasant, seemingly unstoppable worries. It feels like your mind is on a continuously recurring loop, replaying thoughts that are dragging you into the scary future. *What will happen if she doesn't find better friends at school? If she continues to dislike school, will she decide not to go to college? What if she never finds a sense of purpose the rest of her life?*

What are we supposed to do when this happens?

The Stockholm Syndrome

The first step is to grasp what is happening in our minds when we've been ensnared by rumination. Studies of physical hijackings have identified a curious psychological phenomenon among hostages named the "Stockholm syndrome." The term originated from a botched 1973 bank robbery in Sweden where robbers, who were trapped in the bank by the police, held several bank employees and customers as hostages for multiple days. During the kidnapping, a strange thing happened—the hostages psychologically bonded with their captors. The hostages identified so completely with their hijackers that even after their rescue, they publicly defended their captors and raised money for their legal defense.

This pattern has been documented over and over in hijackings, persecutions, and abusive relationships. The Stockholm syndrome is especially pervasive among abused spouses, where the abused cannot imagine a life apart from the abuser. The longer the abduction or abuse lasts, the more the hostages are prone to merging their identity with their oppressors. Stockholm syndrome sufferers don't even recognize that this mental fusion has occurred.

Rumination is a form of the Stockholm syndrome in which anxious thoughts are the hijacker. When we have been mentally abducted by anxiety for extended periods, we identify so thoroughly with the anxious thoughts that our minds fuse with these thoughts. This is why family members and friends of conspiracy theorists report a feeling that some alien being has abducted their loved one. The more we rehearse an anxious narrative, the more we become indistinguishable from the narrative, such that we cannot abandon those thoughts. This mental fusion can be so complete we sometimes don't even recognize that we've been hijacked.

Rumination is the most pervasive and painful symptom of anxiety's hold over our minds, but there is a way out.

The Power of Naming

The Bible ascribes great power to the act of naming. Both Old and New Testaments are filled with narratives where naming people, places, and animals is important. This act is so significant that the first task given to Adam and Eve was to name the other creatures (Genesis 2:18–20). In God's design, to be human is to exercise the power of naming.

Naming is powerful because it establishes two key aspects of the relationship between the namer and the named—differentiation and authority.

Let's start with differentiation. When I name another being, I am recognizing that this being is truly "another." It is not me and hence deserves another name. This is why parents name their newborns at birth. The parent, in the act of naming, recognizes that this baby—who had previously been merged with the mother's body—now exists as a separate, differentiated being.

Similarly, in the creation story, when Eve labeled the four-legged creature standing before her "tiger," she was reminded that this beast was not "Eve." She was not to confuse her identity with this other being. This was an important reminder in the ancient religious context in which the Bible was first written. Pantheism—the belief that all beings and things are merged with one another in ultimate identity—was prevalent then and persists to this day.

Naming also is an exercise of authority. After my pastoral career ended, I eventually began my current consulting company. At the time, it was a scary step to move into the secular world, and I felt insecure about whether I could make my way in this world. I remember when I submitted the official paperwork for incorporation and had to enter the company's name. Empowerment surged through me as I wrote out the name I had come up with. I was exercising authority over my future.

Authority and naming rights are especially intertwined in the biblical tradition. The Israelites exercised their God-given authority over the promised land by naming one patch after another. In the Gospels, when Jesus called his disciples, he gave new nicknames to some—for example, Simon became Peter, "the Rock." Jesus, as the Master, understood the true nature of his disciples and expressed his authority in naming. With Adam and Eve, God was granting them authority over the beasts that roamed Eden through the act of naming them.

As descendants of Adam and Eve, we have been granted this same differentiation and authority vis-à-vis our mental beasts as well. When we can name our thoughts, we recognize them as distinct from us. We are meant to recognize our anxious thoughts as things that may roam in our minds, but they are not "us" in our entirety. There is a critical difference between a thought present within us and a thought becoming us. Anxiety inescapably afflicts the human condition, but we are not meant to bond with our anxiety. Paul's encouragement in Philippians 4:6—"Do not be anxious"—implies it is possible to differentiate ourselves from anxiety. It is possible to "not *be* your anxious thoughts." Anxious thoughts will come, but we do not become them. We can differentiate. You also can recognize that you are not your hijacker.

Naming Anxiety in Our Minds

Naming can help us establish this differentiation in our minds. In my season of parental anxiety, I practiced naming during sessions of mindful breathing. In these sessions, the anxious thoughts would often sneak in and my mind fused with them in rumination. But my mindful breath and repeated prayer reminded me that my true identity is with Jesus, not with those thoughts.

Those spiritual practices served as a stable mental platform from which I could better observe my anxious thoughts. The key was to observe them—with a kind of detached and curious posture—and not to engage with them. We are vulnerable to fusion when we actively engage with those thoughts. Giving actual names to those thoughts help maintain that important differentiation. I started with literal names and shared them with Jesus in prayer: "Oh look, Jesus, there's the 'I must have done something wrong as a parent' thought again."[1]

When I named my anxious thoughts, a fascinating thing happened. I began to experience a sense of authority over them. The more I could stand outside of my anxious thoughts, observe them, and label them, the more those thoughts began to lose their power to terrify. They stopped roaming with impunity like tigers in a jungle. Instead, they became slower, tamer, almost still. I was bringing them under the power of my recognition. The more I watched those thoughts with detached observation and not engagement and the more I said, "Oh, I recognize you," the more the anxious thoughts faded away.

This departure of my anxious thoughts didn't happen right away or every time. When they persisted, it almost always was when I had allowed myself to engage and fuse with the anxious thoughts rather than name them as a detached observer. It takes some practice to stay on the side of detached curiosity without falling into fusion. Many times, I had been watching the tiger-like thoughts from afar, only to realize I had essentially hopped on the back of the tiger and was being carried headlong into a scary future. At that point, the key was to recognize the mental abduction, gently return to the mindful breath (without beating myself up for falling momentarily into the Stockholm syndrome), and resume my observation. I gradually regained my differentiated authority.

One cannot maintain this detached posture throughout a normal day. It is best to set aside some short, dedicated time period to build the mental muscles involved. I deliberately set time aside on thirty-minute walks to imagine my mind as a radio playing broadcasts from different "stations." This was a helpful way to recognize all the different mental streams occurring in my mind. I would give radio call signs to each of these stations I'd pick up on those walks. For example, I had KWORK for thoughts about my consulting practice or KFOOD for my thoughts about lunch (I think *a lot* about the different possibilities for sprucing up my ramen).[2]

I paid particular attention to a station I called KFEAR. I even gave KFEAR an imaginary disc jockey (he had a classic, exaggerated baritone voice like "Dr. Johnny Fever" from a sitcom from my youth, *WKRP in Cincinnati*). With KFEAR, it was especially critical to maintain a differentiated but slightly curious listening posture. When my rumination ramped up, I deliberately said to myself, *Oh, KFEAR is on again. What's it playing now?*

In that season, most of what KFEAR played involved parental anxieties. To help me recognize these soundtracks more quickly, I did more naming. Doing so helped me recognize that KFEAR actually played the same songs over and over, an insight that was illuminating and empowering. Whenever I hopped on the back of my anxious thoughts and galloped into the scary future, my mental world seemed overwhelming in its complexity and rapidly shifting scenes. My mind was a blur. But whenever I stepped into observer mode, I realized how simple KFEAR was. It mostly played two or three tracks over and over again. Everything slowed and became clearer.

Only rarely would I hear a new song—and those can be moments of especially helpful recognition. On one walk, for instance, I picked up a stream of thought I hadn't noticed before. I eventually titled the song "Oh, but What Will the Other Parents Think?" (it had the jaunty feel of an old-time Broadway musical ditty). The discovery startled me at first because I thought I didn't care about that sort of thing. However, that particular thought loop had exercised significant hypnotic power over me precisely by staying hidden to my conscious mind. Naming that song revealed both its presence and also its hidden origins. As a Chinese American, I had witnessed up close how destructive that soundtrack was in my community, and I vowed to not be that kind of parent. It was humbling to realize I carried those lyrics within me. I felt my will strengthening. It motivated me to ask Jesus to deal with this song because I didn't want it to represent my true self.

Bringing Our Internal Voices to Jesus

What does Jesus do with the voices we bring to him? He exercises his differentiation and authority on our behalf. This is beautifully illustrated in one of my favorite gospel stories—the healing of the Gerasene demoniac (Mark 5:1–13). Typical rumination should not be attributed to demonic oppression (although I also cannot rule out some connection in certain cases), but there are some fascinating parallels. Demon possession is the most extreme hijack of a person. It is the most spiritually destructive form of the Stockholm syndrome, where abductees merge their identity almost entirely with the oppressor. Moreover, the scene is shot through with anxiety in both the fears of the Gerasene community and the demon-possessed man's fear-filled cry to Jesus. How Jesus responds to this man provides helpful analogies to the way Jesus responds to our anxiety.

Here is the story:

[Jesus and his disciples] came to the other side of the sea, to the country of the Gerasenes. And when Jesus had stepped out of the boat, immediately there met him out of the tombs a man with an unclean spirit. He lived among the tombs. And no one could bind him anymore, not even with a chain, for he had often been bound with shackles and chains, but he wrenched the chains apart, and he broke the shackles in pieces. No one had the strength to subdue him. Night and day among the tombs and on the mountains he was always crying out and cutting himself with stones. And when he saw Jesus from afar, he ran and fell down before him. And crying out with a loud voice, he said, "What have you to do with me, Jesus, Son of the Most High God? I adjure you by God, do not torment me." For he was saying to him, "Come out of the man, you unclean spirit!" And Jesus asked him, "What is your name?" He replied, "My name is Legion, for we are many." And he begged him earnestly not to send them out of the country. Now a great herd of pigs was feeding there on the hillside, and they begged him, saying, "Send us to the pigs; let us enter them." So he gave them permission. And the unclean spirits came out and entered the pigs; and the herd,

numbering about two thousand, rushed down the steep bank
into the sea and drowned in the sea. (Mark 5:1–13 ESV)

The poor man was so fused with his demonic oppressor that
the two were indistinguishable to his neighbors and even to himself. In Mark 5:7, when the voice cries out, "What have you to do
with me?" it is not at all clear who is the "me" speaking—the man
himself or the demon. But in verse 8, Jesus exercises spiritual
authority to establish differentiation: "Come out of *the man*, you
unclean spirit!" (emphasis added). He insists on a clear distinction between "the man" and the "unclean spirit."

And how is this differentiation and authority expressed most
powerfully? Jesus does not go so far as to name the demon—it
already had a name—but he exercises naming authority by commanding that the name of the oppressor be revealed (Mark 5:9).

"My name is Legion." What a startling answer. Legion
was the name of the basic unit of the Roman army, the force
oppressing the land of Israel at the time (the unit numbered two
thousand men, which explains Mark's inclusion of the number
of pigs listed in Mark 5:13).

There are multiple possible layers to this revelation. Certainly,
this name confirms the biblical worldview that dark spiritual
forces are behind human forms of oppression, and these spiritual
forces can hijack an individual's very identity. Does the revelation
of "Legion" mean this hijacking occurred because this man was
himself a victim of Roman brutality? Or perhaps this man was
one of the many native militants who was obsessively consumed
by a hatred of the Roman invaders, such that over time he had
fused himself with a narrative of violent retribution? In other
words, was he an ancient and extreme version of those today
who have given over their identities to our political conflicts?
We aren't given the full backstory, so these are just conjectures.

In any case, the important fact conveyed by the story is not how this hijacking occurred, but rather that Jesus has the authority to deal with all forms of bondage, whether it be psychological, spiritual, cultural, or political. By himself, the man could not free himself from his mental captivity; this bondage was only revealed by Jesus' exercise of authority. To further dramatize his authority to free humans from our various forms of the Stockholm syndrome, Jesus casts the oppressive Legion into two thousand pigs that disappear over a cliff into the sea.

Imagine the man standing with Jesus. Side by side, they observe the differentiation. The oppressive voices, which had held the man captive for so long that they had become almost indistinguishable from the man himself, are now being separated from him visibly.

It was as if Jesus were pointing to the shrieking swine and saying to the man, "There goes Legion over there. You are here with me. Legion is under my control. You are free." He thus conveys to the man, "You no longer need to be obsessively consumed by this threat."

This is the same Jesus who stands with us in our current bondage to rumination. You can bring to him the anxious voices inside you. With him, you can differentiate from your worries: *There goes my looping thoughts. I am here with Jesus.* He will share his authority with you and reassure you, *Your abductor is under my control. You can go free.*

The process of liberation probably won't involve a scene as dramatic as two thousand pigs rushing off a cliff and drowning in the sea. It may not be as sudden (although it could be). How Jesus will free you will reflect your unique history, wiring, and relationship with him. But whatever the eventual process of liberation looks like, it begins with our willingness to name our anxious self and bring that part of us to Jesus.

The analogy between the demon-possessed Gerasene and our anxiety only goes so far. While specific anxious thoughts can be cast out (often over time), our underlying anxious nature cannot be sent over a cliff and banished forever. Anxiety is part of the human condition. To banish KFEAR entirely is to reject something of my humanity. KFEAR exists within me, and I am more human when I recognize this reality.

However, recognition is not fusion. When I stand with Jesus, I can recognize the anxious voices within me without bonding with those voices. I can observe the thoughts without hopping on their back and letting them carry me into a fearful future. As I asked Jesus to help me in this process, I improved at differentiating those voices in my listening and naming sessions.

Recognition is not fusion.

I'm also growing in confidence in my ability to exercise my God-given authority over anxiety. For people like me who suffer from rumination, it is important to know when to listen and when to change the channel. Listening to our anxiety is helpful when we've decided to set aside the time and are prepared with practices like mindful breathing to anchor ourselves in that detached position with Jesus. Listening to our anxiety is destructive when we need to get our work done, converse with a friend, or parent a child. If we listen to anxiety in situations meant for another purpose, we generally will be too distracted to recognize the hijacker's subtle moves. We will be highly vulnerable to unconsciously fusing with anxiety.

As an expression of my God-given authority in those times meant for other purposes, I imagined on my mental radio a large, old-fashioned set of readings and dials. If I caught myself replaying my worries at an unhelpful time, I envisioned the radio frequency reading as stuck on KFEAR.

"Thanks, KFEAR, but not now," I said, sometimes out loud

if I was alone (don't laugh). "I'll get back to you at our regularly scheduled time." In my mind, I would turn the dial to a channel more appropriate for the activity at hand, like KWORK. Sometimes that other channel was KPRAY—a soundtrack explicitly involving God, such as mindful breathing or listening to a worship song. But at other times, the most helpful practice was to tune to a mental channel playing something pleasantly distracting. For me, it might be tuning to a baseball game (on an actual radio station!). Regardless, I was consciously acknowledging my anxiety and granting it a "station" in my mind but still exercising my God-given differentiation and authority.

This "changing the channel" practice worked sometimes, but not always. Sometimes the KFEAR soundtrack still played loudly on loop. Whenever that happened, I imagined the volume spiking into the red zone. I then tried to imagine myself turning down the volume dial until the soundtrack was a more manageable background murmur. It was my way of giving myself permission to feel some anxiety but still refuse to be carried away entirely.

Naming Anxiety in Our Bodies

Another way to tell whether anxious thoughts are taking over is by listening to your body. Anxiety also reveals itself physically.

While anxiety can lurk unnoticed by our conscious mind, many telltale bodily signs can allow us to grow our recognition skills. Here are some common physical symptoms of anxiety:

- stomach discomfort
- headache
- pounding heart

- rapid breathing
- tight chest
- trouble sleeping
- muscle tension or pain
- trembling or shaking

We can have some or all of these symptoms when we're anxious.

These physical reactions are the product of our body's natural fight-or-flight system. God designed this system so that human beings could respond to real and present threats. Over eons of human existence, this system has served that purpose for us. These instincts are hardwired into our bodies. Our ancestors relied on this bodily system to meet concrete dangers right before them, like a wolf suddenly appearing on the horizon or a fire erupting in a cave dwelling.

All of these symptoms stem from some way our bodies are mobilizing to help us in that real and present moment. For example, let's go back to my eight-year-old latchkey self. Why did I always feel a sinking sensation in the pit of my stomach? It was because my digestive system was shutting down in order to direct maximal blood flow to my large muscle groups. I envisioned a threat, so my body reacted by getting my muscles fully oxygenated to fight a hidden threat. My heart pounded in order to keep my blood flow going.

Or why did I fire my pitches all over the place on the Little League mound? Because I imagined the future and anticipated the shame. I wanted to flee that feeling, so my body tensed my muscles to help me flee a threat. Those tense muscles were incapable of the fluid motions needed for pitching. Ironically, by imagining a future fear I wanted to flee, my body reacted in a way that hastened its arrival.

Anxiety is counterproductive because it causes our body to engage in fight-or-flight mode for an imagined future threat, not a real and present danger. Our muscles are staying in a tense, fully mobilized state, which is why they feel sore. Our stomachs are shut down, which is why we have digestive pain. We remain in a hypervigilant state, which is why we can't sleep.

When we worry, we stay locked in those bodily reactions because we are locked into the future. Because the imagined future is always ahead of us, our bodies stay locked in the fight-or-flight mode continually, long past what they can sustain healthily.

In other words, while anxiety hijacks your mind into the future, it also hijacks your body into the future. Anxiety is commandeering your natural fight-or-flight system for its "Not Yetness" when God designed it just for his Now.

The more we pay attention to those bodily symptoms, the faster we will recognize anxiety as something happening inside us. This recognition can then alert us to take steps to get present, especially steps that involve some bodily dimension such as getting present to nature and mindful breathing.

Naming Anxiety in Our Relationships

Physical symptoms—such as a two-week period of insomnia—force us to pay attention and recognize our own inner anxiety. But anxiety can sometimes stay below the threshold of recognizable physical symptoms. We may also need to pay attention to the way anxiety is present in our relationships.

The same fight-or-flight system that commandeers our minds and bodies can also take over our relationships. Here are some common ways that anxiety shows up in our behavior with others:

Fight	Flight
TOWARD THE THREAT	AWAY FROM THE THREAT
Insistent and aggressive	Deferring and passive
Critical and irritated with others	Self-critical and self-blaming
	Paralyzed
Jumpy and flitting	Sad
Angry	Quiet
Loud	Resistant to change
Demanding immediate action	Hiding
Putting self forth	Watching cat videos
Obsessively consuming news, charts, opinions of experts	

Every individual can engage in both sides of this chart. Each of us can flip back and forth between fight or flight in relationships, but we tend to lean one way or another. Can you use this chart to locate your tendency?

The key is to connect these behaviors with underlying anxiety, with the fight-or-flight response happening "in here." This is a challenging ask, because as I've already pointed out, we are tempted to explain these behaviors as something happening "out there." When we deflect blame "out there," we can damage our relationships—because the target "out there" is often a loved one.

Let me give you an example. I lean pretty heavily in the "fight" mode when I get anxious. My wife, Jody, tends to lean more toward the "flight" side.

Around the time the COVID-19 crisis hit, I received a medical diagnosis of a heart condition that put me at a higher risk of complications if I were to contract the virus. This awareness naturally made me even more anxious.

As a "fight" person, I swung into a mode of heading toward the threat. I did marathon Google searches on my condition. I bought devices to monitor my heart. All of these steps led to even more questions. A doctor friend at church agreed to answer my questions, so I asked Jody if she would join me in the phone call.

Now here's where my inability to recognize my anxiety comes in. Or perhaps I should say, my inability to let others recognize my anxiety. I did not tell my wife what I was feeling. If I had been willing to share with her, I would have said something like, "Honey, I'm anxious about what's going on and would be reassured if you were by my side when we talked to the doctor on the phone."

Instead, what I said to her was this: "Look, I don't want to have to repeat all the same information for you, and I want you to be able to ask her your questions." Notice again the subtle pushing "out there" to make this request be about Jody and her needs—not about my inner anxiety.

Jody tends to head away from intractable problems (such as my medical diagnosis) toward other tasks she can control. The night of our scheduled phone call with the doctor, she was trying to knock out her shopping list at three different stores. Her last stop was Target. Buying supplies was for her a manageable and unthreatening task—different from both COVID-19 and my medical condition. So right before our scheduled time with the doctor, she called me and said she would call in from the aisles of Target.

I got angry, but in a pouty, passive-aggressive way.

"Fine. Sure." I get monosyllabic when I'm hurt. "If that's what you want to do, if it's *that* important to you to finish your shopping. Make sure you mute yourself when Target announces the special on laundry detergent."

My hostility confused Jody. She thought I cared about her getting all the information so I didn't have to repeat things to her. She felt she could accomplish that by calling in, and she wanted to check toilet paper off her list. She felt angry with my passive-aggressive hostility.

Neither of us could recognize our underlying anxiety. I was in fight mode, and she was in flight mode—and we were missing each other. I misinterpreted her "flight" behavior as a lack of care. She understood my "fight" behavior as unwarranted hostility, not as a cry for shared presence. We hurt each other out of unrecognized anxiety.

Recognition is so very important. Unrecognized anxiety hijacks our minds, our bodies, and even our most important relationships.

The Growth Opportunity in Relationships

While anxiety can cause damage, it can also be used by God to unlock lasting growth. This opportunity exists in our relationships as well, especially as we grow in the practice of recognition.

My wife and I have been realizing that some of our marital conflicts are driven by the underlying difference in our respective fight-or-flight reactions. A particularly challenging aspect of this process involves recognizing our different reactions as morally neutral. Neither is a sin. Nor is one reaction intrinsically better than the other. We need both because sometimes it is better to flee from the wolf and sometimes we've got to fight the fire. But as a hijacker of relationships, anxiety deviously cloaks itself in moral clothing. When we don't recognize a common anxiety underneath differing reaction patterns, we lock in on surface differences and place a **Anxiety cloaks itself in moral clothing.** moral label on them. We judge and blame the other. The fight person labels the flight person as "lazy" or "inattentive." The flight person labels the fight person as "rude" or "nagging."[3]

Relational growth through anxiety involves helping the other person recognize what is really happening and then finding common ground in the underlying anxiety. Jody and I have even developed shorthand codes for this. In the middle of some conflict where we're labeling and judging the other's response pattern, Jody may suddenly realize what's going on (and she's better at this than I am). She will get a twinkle in her eye, give me a sly smile, and pump her arms up and down in a running motion. It's her disarmingly funny way of signaling, *Okay, I admit it. I'm anxious, and I'm fleeing here!* And the conflict de-escalates. We find common ground in a shared anxiety. I can recognize and admit I'm in fight mode. We're able to empathize with each other and even chuckle at ourselves.

There is something remarkable about people who are collectively growing their ability to recognize anxiety. That's because emotion is contagious—it can spread from one person to another. Psychologists call this phenomenon "social contagion."

This can be *good*. Have you ever been in an antisocial mood, which then disappeared when you walked into a festive party? Suddenly you're more ebullient, with more of a pep in your step?

It can be *neutral*. When someone yawns, laughs, or smiles in your presence and you find yourself doing the same thing in response, this is the involuntary "catching" of behaviors and attitudes across connected individuals.[4]

But it can be *bad*, as stockbrokers know all too well. Wall Street's "Fear Index" is based on the reality that collective fear can cause stocks to trade below their value. In fact, the collective anxiety of stockholders can cause entire markets to crash.

You may have personally felt the negative form of social contagion acutely during the COVID-19 pandemic when one quick conversation with a worried individual put you into an emotional tailspin. With the proliferation of social media, you don't even have to be in the same room with the affected persons to catch it.

In other words, our emotions affect others in mysterious but significant ways. That's why it is important to think seriously about your anxiety, because whether you know it or not, it is affecting others in your company, your friendship group, and your family.

My professional life is now focused on seeking the health of entire organizations. My clients are mostly secular nonprofits and government agencies, and I now coach many CEOs and train emerging leaders of these organizations. Because of the way anxiety ended my own career as a leader in a church, I'm especially tuned in to the presence of anxiety in the organizational leaders I serve and the ways they can act as powerful super-spreaders of anxiety.

One of my most consistently impactful interventions is helping them see how their anxiety can drive their management practices. My CEOs tend to have high-functioning anxiety, like I do. Also like me, they tend to default to fight mode. They often plunge forward with their own versions of firing off long emails to their staff at three in the morning. Too often, their colleagues don't push back. Team members don't realize their leader's behavior is anxiety-driven. Instead, they feel confused, insecure, guilty, and blamed. Anxiety spreads like a contagion throughout the entire organization.

Anxiety spreads most viciously when it remains unnamed. This is true for an individual person, and it is especially true for an organization. Sadly, leaders of organizations are not taught or encouraged to recognize and name their own anxiety. Every year, I instruct a cohort of emerging leaders, individuals who have been selected because they'll likely be the future CEOs in my sector. These people have almost always received prior training on how to track key issues on their balance sheet or performance metrics. Every year, I ask them if any of them have received training on how to spot anxiety in their own leadership. No one has ever raised their hand.

My cohort program reserves an entire day to help them recognize their anxiety as a doorway for growth. When they walk through that door, they begin to unlock their best self as a leader. I've seen this kind of growth in self-awareness in the leaders when they can admit to their staff something like, "Hey, what's going on for me right now is I'm anxious we're not going to make our fundraising targets this year and I'll look bad with the board." A simple admission like this unlocks profound growth in organizational cultures. Conflict de-escalates. Compassion grows. People chip in to help. Everyone learns to laugh at themselves a bit. And those organizational values, which grew out of a simple recognition of anxiety, end up blossoming in other areas as well.

That's the beauty of the Anxiety Opportunity.

CHAPTER 6

Accepting Our Anxious Self

W alt Whitman's 1855 poem "Song of Myself" makes a famous observation. "Do I contradict myself? Very well then I contradict myself," he wrote. "I am large, I contain multitudes."[1]

What are those multitudes?

Psychologists used to believe we all had mono-minds, that we could dig deeply enough to reveal a singular true inner self. Now, however, they believe we're much more complicated. It seems the best way to understand our psyches is as a composition of different parts. In a sense, we contain different "selves" that feel, want, and avoid different things. This psychological insight was captured in the Pixar movie *Inside Out*, which dramatized these different selves as actual characters interacting—and sometimes fighting—with each other inside the heroine's mind.

This internal dialogue happens constantly. Right now, a part of me as the author of this book thinks this chapter intro is wonderful; another part is criticizing myself as a hack; another part of me is telling me to finish it already; and yet another part of me wants to go eat ramen. My different parts can, as Whitman put it, "contradict myself."

If you similarly paused in the middle of some decision-making process, you would also recognize your own version of your multitudes. You might even be able to identify some of those voices. Perhaps you, too, hear a "critic self" telling you you're not good enough (a voice that, for some, sounds awfully similar to the voice of a particularly hard-to-please parent), another "cheerleader self" pumping you up ("You got this!"), another "calculator self" coolly tabulating pros and cons, and so on and so on.

Modern psychologists weren't the first to recognize this "multiple selves" truth. The Bible describes this reality. In Matthew 22:37, Jesus cites the ancient wisdom of Deuteronomy 6:5 in stating the greatest commandment as "love the Lord your God with all your heart and with all your soul and with all your mind." The commandment assumes the structure of at least three distinct "selves"—a "heart" self, a "soul" self, and a "mind" self. Even within each particular self, there is the possibility of further division such that the emphasis on *all* is needed with each one.

Moreover, the Bible sometimes depicts these different internal aspects as characters interacting with each other. Take, for example, Psalm 103:1–2 (ESV): "Bless the LORD, O my soul, and all that is within me, bless his holy name! Bless the LORD, O my soul, and forget not all his benefits." The author is instructing his "soul" to join in with the rest of his internal multitudes ("all that is within me") in praising God—which, again, implies the potential of disagreement among these distinct selves.

While the "heart, soul, mind" structure is a common way the Bible depicts the inner multitudes, it is not the only way the Bible does so. The Bible elsewhere suggests the possibility of other depictions. For instance, in Romans 7, Paul describes at length two different parts of his inner being as different "laws" engaged in battle. He poignantly describes the agony of this inner strife: "For in my inner being I delight in God's law; but I see another law at work in me, waging war against the law of my mind and making me a prisoner of the law of sin at work within me. What a wretched man I am!" (7:22–24). According to Paul, the contradiction within our "multitudes" that Walt Whitman described can escalate into outright bullying. What is more important than any one scheme is this underlying insight that we have distinct inner selves that can be in conflict with each other.

Understanding—and healing—this inner conflict is the next step in the Anxiety Opportunity.

Our Anxious Self

Our Anxious Self is a complex member of our inner multitudes. Sometimes it is the bully, like when it hijacks us into the future. But our Anxious Self can also be the one getting bullied. We often don't like our Anxious Self at all.

For most of my life, I rejected mine. In fact, I hated it. My Anxious Self felt weak and scared. I didn't like that worried eight-year-old who called his mom's office. I cringed at the memory of that Little Leaguer bursting into tears coming off the mound. I hated that insomniac senior pastor who stared at the ceiling for hours, ruminating about the budget and staff conflicts. I had contempt for my Anxious Self cowering in the parking lot of the pumpkin patch while my family picked out their future jack-o'-lanterns.

Search back in your memory and bring to mind your version of my eight-year-old latchkey kid or my Little Leaguer struggling on the mound. Perhaps you can more readily summon an even more recent experience, perhaps from work or within the context of a relationship. As you contemplate yourself in that memory, how do you feel about your Anxious Self? Do you cringe? Do you stand off in judgment? Do you feel an impulse to look away, wishing that part of your self didn't exist?

Or do you feel drawn to your Anxious Self? Do you reach out in compassion and acceptance? This chapter explores the *acceptance* of our Anxious Self. Why is that acceptance so important? Our inner anxiety is a key context for spiritual growth. Jesus meets us "in here," with our Anxious Self. If we reject our Anxious Self, we are rejecting the presence of Jesus. We are turning away from the place where he wishes to meet us.

In a real sense, accepting Jesus requires accepting our Anxious Self.

Many of us struggle with this step. When encountering our Anxious Self, we are tempted to reject this part of our self and may even feel a degree of self-hatred.

Why do we find our Anxious Selves so unacceptable? Why do so many of us feel revulsion?

I rejected my Anxious Self because I had another version of myself inside me. Let's call this version my Ideal Self. My Ideal Self is the image I want to project to the world. It is how I want others to view me.

My Ideal Self wants to appear strong, not weak. My Ideal Self wants to appear confident, not scared. My Ideal Self wants to appear calm, not sleepless with worry.

Our Anxious Self often presents itself as the complete opposite of our Ideal Self. To the Ideal Self, the Anxious Self can seem like an ugly, disgusting beast, so the Ideal Self compels us to reject our Anxious Self.

For many people, this battle between our Ideal Self and our Anxious Self goes on all the time. For much of my life, my Ideal Self won the battle. So I obeyed my Ideal Self and tried to put the Anxious Self out of view. I banished that ugly creature to the basement of my mind.

But even if it is rejected and banished out of view, the Anxious Self does not disappear. Why? Because the Anxious Self is an unavoidable part of our self.

Remember, anxiety is part of being human, of being "Now and Not Yet" creatures. In naming practices such as my interactions with KFEAR, it is important to still grant anxiety a place on the dial—even as we may purposely turn the dial whenever listening to that particular self is not helpful in a given moment.

The Anxious Self is an unavoidable part of our self. Anxiety is part of being human.

We cannot successfully banish our Anxious Self. The Anxious Self is part of us, so it will always figure out a way to be acknowledged. It will devise some way out of the basement. Sometimes it will sneak out via an otherwise harmless phone call to a bank. Other times it will burst out and wreak havoc on a career. Even if our Ideal Self insists on banishment, our Anxious Self won't go away.

We have to figure out how to get to acceptance.

Jesus and the Anxious Leper

Our secular culture greatly values "self-acceptance." But "self-acceptance" is hampered by a major limitation. In the secular version of "self-acceptance," there is only the "self" in the picture. There is only the self around to do the accepting.

What happens if there is a battle going on inside one's self? And what if one especially strong version of your self—your Ideal Self—absolutely does not want to do any accepting? My Ideal Self is so strong that I need someone else—other than me—to do the accepting. I need someone else in the picture.

This is where we need Jesus in the picture—the one who is depicted in so many stories in the Gospels as the one who welcomes anxious people. One such story is found in Mark 1:40–45, the story of a man who had leprosy. Though short, the story is packed with great meaning, and it is worth your time to read it imaginatively:

> And a leper came to him, imploring him, and kneeling said to him, "If you will, you can make me clean." Moved with pity, he stretched out his hand and touched him and said to him, "I will; be clean." And immediately the leprosy left him, and he was made clean. And Jesus sternly charged him and sent him away at once, and said to him, "See that you say nothing to anyone, but go, show yourself to the priest and offer for your cleansing what Moses commanded, for a proof to them." But he went out and began to talk freely about it, and to spread the news, so that Jesus could no longer openly enter a town, but was out in desolate places, and people were coming to him from every quarter. (Mark 1:40–45 ESV)

The story begins in verse 40: "And a leper came to him, imploring him. . . ." The verb *imploring* (or *begging*, as some translations have it) comes up frequently in Mark and implies emotional distress. But we don't even need to see that verb in this verse to recognize the leper as a deeply anxious person.

In that society, a leper would have lived with constant health anxiety, as he daily checked his skin to see if the leprosy was spreading and worsening. He would have lived with constant financial anxiety, as lepers could not work and could only beg for their food. And he would have lived with constant interpersonal anxiety, as lepers were considered unclean, forbidden to come into close contact with others. Everyone recoiled from lepers, disgusted by their blemished skin. Some lepers suffered from deformed limbs, giving them even more hideous appearances. In every way, a leper was a person banished to the basement of society, to be kept hidden out of view. The leper represents what the Anxious Self is like for our Ideal Selves today.

Look now at the way Jesus responds differently. Jesus is "moved with pity" (Mark 1:41). Jesus feels love and affection for the Anxious Self. Jesus has sympathy and understanding for the Anxious Self. And Jesus communicates his feelings in a way that, for the leper, was more powerful than words. Jesus "stretched out his hand and touched him" (v. 41). Imagine what that must have felt like for the leper. Everyone else recoiled from him in disgust. Jesus alone reached out to touch him. Jesus did what no one else was willing to do. Jesus radically accepted the Anxious Self.

Notice when this acceptance takes place in the order of events. Jesus stretches out his hand to touch the leper *before* the healing. Jesus accepts the leper in his anxious state before he removes the anxiety-producing conditions. The leper is not first "made right" and then acceptance is offered. The acceptance comes first.

As we will see, the leper is not going to "do right," even after the acceptance is granted. The acceptance is given, even though there is the real possibility (which turns out to actually happen) of future disobedience of Jesus' commands. Jesus' acceptance is unconditional. The welcome stands, regardless of the leper's eventual disobedience.

Let that sink in. Jesus accepts our Anxious Self before he heals our anxiety. Jesus accepts you as your Anxious Self, not after you get rid of your anxiety. Jesus accepts you even if you are going to keep messing up. Jesus accepts you unconditionally.

The question for us is, "Will we go along? Will we receive Jesus' acceptance of our Anxious Self? Will we take him up on his offer?" True "self-acceptance" is accepting Jesus' prior and complete acceptance of us—all of us.

What about the Ideal Self? What about the version of you that battles and hates and rejects your Anxious Self? Well, believe it or not, Jesus also accepts your Ideal Self. But your Ideal Self is not the Lord of your life. Jesus is. Your Ideal Self does not get to call the shots. Jesus does. So if Jesus accepts your Anxious Self, your Ideal Self needs to go along.

This process of accepting Jesus' acceptance takes time. Initially, the best I could do was to get my Ideal Self out of the way and allow Jesus to have his way. My Ideal Self would go sulk in the corner and kind of roll his eyes at how Jesus was tenderly receiving my Anxious Self. My Ideal Self was sort of muttering, *Why is Jesus hanging out with this idiot?*

But over time, Jesus has been drawing my Ideal Self from its corner and has been touching that part of me as well. My Ideal Self is learning to be more like Jesus. My Ideal Self is becoming more like Jesus in feeling compassionate about my weaker parts. My Ideal Self is learning to reach out toward—and to accept—my Anxious Self.

That internal acceptance is spiritual growth. It makes me more whole. It brings peace to the internal battle between my Ideal Self and my Anxious Self. This wholeness and peace allows my Ideal Self—how I want others to view me—to include my Anxious Self. My Ideal Self has things to learn from my Anxious Self. The two parts are meant to live together, to grow together.

I don't have to banish my Anxious Self to the basement. I can compassionately introduce to others my "worried eight-year-old" self, my "sleepless senior pastor" self, my "husband in fight mode" self. I'm introducing those selves to you now; in fact, I've never shared those stories in print before now. It has taken years of spiritual growth to get to this point. Spiritual growth takes time, but it increasingly makes me whole. The Anxiety Opportunity provides the chance for you to realize your version of this wholeness as well.

Take a moment to review how you feel about this part of yourself. Are you willing to ask your Ideal Self to stop the war against your Anxious Self? Will you grant the latter a home inside yourself? Can you envision Jesus stretching out his hand toward your Anxious Self? What is Jesus saying to your Anxious Self? And just as importantly, as this happens, what is Jesus saying to your Ideal Self?

Skipping the Growth

Jesus' desire for us to become whole people is conveyed in the concluding details of the story of the man who had leprosy. In Mark 1:43–44, Jesus charges the leper to introduce himself to others. The introduction begins, naturally enough, with the leper's presentation of himself to the priest. The priest was the keeper of "the Ideal" for that society. The priestly system initially banished the leper, but it also certified the healing so others could confidently restore relationships with him. Jesus desires for the leper to be made truly whole and to experience a fuller acceptance.

As I mentioned, the leper disobeys Jesus and skips this next stage of spiritual growth. He was so excited about his newfound relief that he didn't think he needed anything more. So he lost his Anxiety Opportunity, his next step toward more lasting transformation. In doing so, the leper not only cut short his own restoration but also threw a wrench into Jesus' larger plans (Mark 1:45). There is in the story's ending a sense of missed opportunity all around.

The unsettling end of this otherwise touching story should serve as a sober heads-up for our own anxiety journey. The leper story is a cautionary tale about the limitations of the "anxiety as irrelevant to spiritual growth" approach, which views anxiety solely as a mental health condition for secular medicine to relieve.

As I've said, no conflict exists between medically delivered relief and spiritual growth. Scripture tells us the presence of Jesus can be found in the restoration of "all things" (Colossians 1:17). Therefore, I'm convinced Jesus acts through secular mental health and many of its approaches, including antianxiety medication. I myself have benefited from such medication and thank Jesus for those drugs. Such relief from anxiety is a good gift from God—period. In general, I do not believe antianxiety medication intrinsically prevents spiritual growth in any way. But they are also not the same. Symptomatic relief from anxiety does not automatically equal spiritual growth.

The story of the leper warns us that we can receive some immediate relief from our anxiety (whether via medication or some other treatment) but pass up the opportunity for the deeper growth Jesus intends. For me, the process of reconciliation between my Ideal Self and my Anxious Self happened after the initial recovery from the worst symptoms. This deeper healing required a growth process that continued years after the worst of my anxiety symptoms had passed. Deeper growth was not a given. I could have paid no attention to it. And it didn't come packaged in a pill. It required listening to Jesus as he prescribed his next growth steps that were custom-designed for me.

What might be Jesus' next prescription for you?

CHAPTER 7

Your Acceptance Move

I'm sitting on my therapist's couch, recounting how I have gotten hijacked yet again. I describe how this unresolved worry in my consulting practice had kept turning over and over in my head, distracting me from enjoying a weekend getaway with my family.

When I finally reach a stopping point, my therapist leans forward with her elbows on her knees and poses her question.

"When you get like that, Curtis, is there is a different move you can make?"

I let out a groan. "I know, I know! I should stop ruminating, but I'm stuck!" I ball up my fist and pound my thigh in frustration. "Argghh, it's like I can't think about anything else."

"I'm not talking about *thinking* differently," she replied gently. "I'm talking about a different *physical* move you can make."

I fall silent, and my fist slows its drumbeat against my thigh. I don't know how to answer. I'm not even totally sure I understand her question.

She senses my confusion and explains. "Curtis, what I'm

asking is this: When you get stuck like this in your head, is there something you can do to get into your body?"

My therapist straightens up suddenly, pauses for a moment, and starts to feel her forearm. "Oh, I'm getting that tingly feeling, Curtis."

I've come to deeply trust many things about my therapist—her perceptive wisdom, her warm compassion for me, and also this one quirky trait. When she senses that we're on the verge of an important breakthrough, she feels a goose-bumpy sensation in her arms. As a highly analytical person, I thought this was weird at first. But years of working with her have taught me the value of paying attention to her body signals.

And in a sense, she was inviting me now to pay closer attention to my own body.

What did my body want to tell me?

Getting Out of Our Heads

Everyone suffers from some anxiety, but the people most vulnerable tend to be those who live mostly in their heads. Anxiety feeds on our minds. It consumes the flow of thoughts in our heads and then loops them in the recursive patterns of rumination. It ratchets up the internal conversation of our inner multitudes and recasts it into a battle between our Ideal Self and our Anxious Self. As we invest ever more of our energy into our minds, we can be inadvertently resupplying our hijacker.

Indeed, one likely causal factor behind the long-term increase of anxiety in our society is the extent to which mental labor has replaced physical labor in the workforce. I am a consultant—my work almost entirely takes place in my head. The internet and smartphones have made us even more stationary creatures of the mind, beings who process the stream of bits on our screens even when we aren't working. We are more anxious because we are moving less.

This is why a large body of research shows that a highly effective way to lower anxiety is to simply increase physical activity. One major study discovered that a physically active lifestyle is associated with up to 60 percent lower risk of developing an anxiety disorder.[1] It is likely that more intense activity generates some of its benefits through physiological effects (such as generating positive hormonal changes), but some meaningful part of the benefit is simply diverting energy from the head to the body. This is why even low-intensity physical activities—such as creating art or playing music—have been shown to reduce anxiety.[2] When we do something good with our bodies, we are less likely to be beating up on ourselves in our minds.

There are many other good options to get out of our heads, including the practices of getting present to nature and mindful breathing discussed earlier. If you feel stuck in your own anxiety, pay attention to what your body might be wanting to do. What moves can you make?

Moving toward Others

One particular type of movement you should especially consider is that of moving toward others. In the last chapter, we learned of how Jesus moved toward the anxious leper by stretching out his hand and touching him. Jesus' move was meant to trigger the leper's own motion to those around him, which is why Jesus ordered the leper to go to the priest for certification of healing, which in turn would free the leper to return to his community, which in turn would allow others to touch this man once again.

Jesus already knew what brain researchers are only recently being able to prove—namely, that engaging in physical touch lowers anxiety. For example, one study squeezed participants inside a tubular MRI machine and subjected them to all sorts of stressful sensations, including unpredictable (but presumably low-level) electric shocks. Participants were given different kinds of access to touch during this anxious experience, ranging from being able to touch a loved one, someone known but somewhat estranged, a complete stranger, or no one at all. Meanwhile, the regions of their brain most associated with anxiety were being measured for neurological activity.

Not surprisingly, those who could touch a loved one recorded the lowest anxiety measurements. Being able to touch someone estranged was better than touching a complete stranger. And the most anxious? Those who could touch no one at all.[3]

We were created to touch others when anxious. This is why Jesus wants anxious people to move their bodies toward others. It seems that when Jesus seeks to change us, he doesn't want this change to remain stuck just in our heads. He wants us to make that change real by expressing it in our relationships—and often in bodily fashion. This was the point of Jesus' parable of the unforgiving servant (see Matthew 18:23–34). The master forgives the debt of his servant and relieves his financial anxiety. But this relief cannot just stay in the man's head. What is in the mind is meant to be expressed by the body.

The parable cleverly reveals the mind of the servant by dramatizing his physical actions with others. He beat up others who suffer the same financial anxiety, as he "grabbed . . . and began to choke" another servant who owed him money (Matthew 18:28). Seeing this, the master revoked the original forgiveness. Instead of mirroring his master's acceptance, the servant had distorted it into a harsh rejection of others. The servant's failure to make the proper next move reveals that the original relief was never truly realized in the servant's mind.

We are meant to move, and to move toward others. God created us as embodied beings relating to other embodied beings. We are not meant to just live in our heads by ourselves. What we wish to be true inside us is meant to be realized physically, and especially in how we relate to those around us. This is basic to all forms of spiritual growth. We love others out of the love we received from Jesus (John 13:34). We serve others out of the ways we have been served by our Lord (Mark 10:43–45). We are made in God's image (Genesis 1:27), which means we grow into our true destiny when we mirror God's character to one another. Jesus conveyed this dynamic of replication via agricultural metaphors (as he so often did in his teaching). In parables like that of the sower (Mark 4:1–10), Jesus explained that the "good soil" provides for the bearing of a good crop. We can only keep growing to the extent we reproduce what was initially seeded in us.

Let's apply this truth back to anxiety. In the same way that Jesus compassionately reached out and accepted the anxious leper, he now reaches out and accepts your Anxious Self. But this acceptance is not meant to just stay in your head.

In the same way that Jesus prescribed actions for the anxious leper to replicate this acceptance in his relationships, Jesus invites us to mirror his acceptance in our relationships. This means that the other Anxious Selves around us are necessary for our own spiritual growth. Anxious people around us are opportunities for us to reflect Jesus' acceptance.

This isn't easy. It requires the ongoing and often hard work of obeying Jesus' instructions to accept one another. This is still true for me. You would think that I—someone who has suffered from anxiety—would naturally be filled with compassion for other anxious people. Nope. Like the unforgiving servant who beat up another servant just like him, I am highly prone to reject other anxious people.

We reject in others what we most reject in ourselves. The Anxious Self in other people reminds me of the Anxious Self in me. So instead of mirroring Jesus' acceptance to others, I engage in my version of the servant's grabbing and choking—not with that level of extreme violence, of course, but in more subtle moves of rejection. It may be an ever so slight roll of my eyes when I listen to a speaker who is struggling with nerves. Or it may be my exasperated sigh when I sense an employee is feeling insecure about an assignment I've just given him—or maybe I'll be able to hide my frustration with him then and there, but when I get home, I let it out in private rants with my wife.

This "dark mirroring" often happens at an unconscious level, but you can learn how to spot it in yourself. Pay attention to the feelings of judgment and revulsion you feel toward others. Other people's anxiety can trigger these feelings in me in a way that doesn't happen with other forms of human frailty. And that's when I know the Holy Spirit is whispering, "Curtis, you need to do some more acceptance work." I've found my next Anxiety Opportunity.

Remember, we dislike in others what we most dislike in ourselves. This dark-mirroring dynamic explains why, in my experience as a consultant, so many CEOs and other seemingly successful leaders have the hardest time accepting anxiety in the people they manage. For example, I've worked with a leader who rose to the top because of her "high-functioning anxiety." Some part of her leadership energy is a sophisticated expression of her fight mode. One particular person on her senior management team especially triggers her. This CEO is still early in her anxiety journey, so she views this person as a real headache, an external problem "out there" (and she wants me to "fix" him). She doesn't recognize that her colleague is mirroring her own anxiety "in here"—anxiety that she hates in herself.

The anxious people in our lives present growth opportunities for us. They serve as pointers to where Jesus' acceptance is still needed in us. Jesus may even now be bringing to mind some anxious person in your life who especially triggers you. If so, you've found your next move.

The Anxious Parent

One person especially needs this prescription—the parent of an anxious child.

Teens have higher levels of anxiety than adults, according to the National Institute of Mental Health (NIMH). A 2021 study demonstrated that while 19 percent of all American adults had suffered from anxiety disorder during that year, anxiety disorder had affected almost 32 percent of teens during that same year. Teen girls suffer from anxiety disorders more than anyone else—a whopping 38 percent compared to 26 percent of male adolescents. And these statistics are only climbing.[4] More than half of Gen Zers say that "they expect the worst to happen."[5] Large-scale studies of thousands of youth show that the average anxiety level of a young person now exceeds the levels recorded by hospitalized psychiatric patients in the 1950s.[6]

One longtime Boston-area pediatrician told my friend, "I used to deal with cuts, scrapes, and bruises, but my practice has morphed into a full-time effort to battle mental issues." The epidemic of youth anxiety is spreading rapidly and is seemingly without end.

Any suffering in children will naturally trigger anxiety in a parent. But there can be an extra jolt when suffering comes in the form of childhood or adolescent anxiety. Given that so much of a parent's Anxious Self was formed by one's own early experiences, seeing anxiety in our children can be like peering into that dark mirror. Your anxious child is likely triggering your own Anxious Childhood Self.

If you still hate what you see in yourself, contempt will likely leak out in your parenting in any number of ways. It could be in the form of judgment, irritation, impatience, guilt, fear, and other feelings that have an extra charge of emotion. Like CEOs replicating anxiety in their organizational system, these parental responses can further heighten anxiety in the family system.

I know that pointing out this dark-mirroring dynamic is going to make some parents feel bad. Parents who are already anxious about their parenting will be tempted to groan and mutter to themselves, *Oh, great, one more thing I have to worry about doing wrong!* Anxious parents might be anxious about feeling anxious, and now (especially after reading this) they'll feel even more anxious that their anxiety will make their children more anxious, which will in turn make them as parents feel even more anxious, and so on and so forth. This is the devious nature of anxiety's dark mirror. When we are mirroring only our Anxious Selves back and forth to each other in our relationships, we end up trapped in one of those Halloween fun house of mirrors that reflect distortion upon distortion.

This is precisely why everything has to start with Jesus' acceptance of us. We need a different mirror, one pointed at Jesus, not at our Self. He must be in the picture as the originating image.

True God-imaging parenting thus starts with the parents themselves receiving God's acceptance. For parents, this means your parenting anxiety is a profound opportunity for your own spiritual growth. Your parenting struggle is where you can receive Jesus' acceptance of you. He embraces all of you, with all of your frailty, failings, and fears as a parent. Even before you've gotten everything right. Even after you keep messing things up. He accepts the Anxious Parent in you.

Because God accepts every anxious parent unconditionally, every parent can mirror God's unconditional acceptance to their children. This parental mirror is fundamentally different from anxiety's dark, fun-house mirroring. It is different because it doesn't start with the Self, and it doesn't involve bouncing back and forth

Jesus accepts the Anxious Parent in you.

with other Anxious Selves. This mirror starts with the picture of Jesus as he is depicted in his unconditional acceptance of the man who had leprosy and so many other hurting people in the Gospels.

As parents, we were designed to serve as a faithful mirror of God. Our parenting is meant to reflect how God parents us (Ephesians 5:1–2). Just as God does, we parents provide instructions, rules, and moral clarity. And just as we often ignore God's instructions, rules, and moral clarity (as the leper did), our children will often ignore ours. But none of that changes the truth that Jesus is standing before us, reaching out to embrace us. His acceptance comes first and foremost. We are accepted by God "while we were still sinners" (Romans 5:8). So our primary job as parents is to reflect radical acceptance to our children as faithfully as we can.

A faithful mirror is not a perfect mirror. Think of a cracked and cloudy mirror—and by the way, the mirrors of the biblical era were often cracked and much cloudier than our modern manufactured ones (see 1 Corinthians 13:12). This kind of mirror does not provide a perfect, crystal clear replica of the source image. But it still faithfully reflects something of the essence. Your parenting is undoubtedly cracked and cloudy in a thousand ways, but in the end, you can mirror the essence of God's radical acceptance to your anxious children. This is your most important task.

Being the parent of an anxious child is an unavoidably bewildering and emotional experience. And even apart from our own emotional struggles, we're confronted with the confusing, practical questions about how we can provide our children with the help they need. We may wonder about such things as professional therapy, types of medication, and dosages.

I'm not a medical professional, so I cannot provide any clarity on these medical fronts. But I can say one thing with absolute certainty. There's one highly effective intervention only you can deliver in a dosage more potent than any secular medical professional could deliver: you can provide acceptance. Radical, loving, compassionate acceptance. The "Jesus touching the leper" kind of acceptance. The acceptance that is expressed with hugs, reassuring pats, and sometimes just the kind of silent but loving physical presence of a parent that anxious children can feel in their bones.

No antianxiety drug is more powerful for a child than the receiving of radical acceptance from parents.

Every parent can receive and deliver this acceptance from our Father God, available to us through Jesus. There is no educational level, income, special skill, licensing, or application required. You are already accepted.

Discovering Your Acceptance Move

To say it one more time, our capacity to accept others' Anxious Selves rests on the prior reality that Jesus has accepted our own Anxious Self. Our acceptance of others organically grows out of Jesus' loving acceptance of us. And therefore we need some way to remind ourselves that we are like that anxious leper who met Jesus somewhere in Galilee.

How do we do this? How do *you* do this—especially if you're someone who also gets stuck in your head?

And now we're back to the moment my therapist asked me, "When you get like that, Curtis, is there is a move you can make?"

I sat on the couch in puzzled silence. I could hear the clock ticking. The rhythmic pounding of my thigh had come to a complete halt. My therapist smiled with a certain calmness, which I knew meant she wasn't going to supply the answer for me.

I tried to quiet my thoughts. I sensed I could not reason or analyze my way to the right move, and so I just tuned into what my body was hungering for.

My right fist released into an open palm. It slowly stretched across my body, reaching toward my left shoulder. The movement was unconscious, as if guided by an outside force. My right hand came to rest on that opposite shoulder, and I gently patted myself, mixing in soft squeezes.

My therapist let out a small little breath and her eyes started to mist. My own vision blurred.

Then I heard myself whisper quietly to myself, *It's all right, kiddo. It's all right.*

"Kiddo"? No one has ever called me "kiddo"—not my parents or anyone else I can remember. Where did that come from?

I believe it came from Jesus. And that "kiddo"? I think he is eight years old.

CHAPTER 8

The Anxiety Formula

The loan officer pushed another stack of documents across the mahogany desk. Before I picked up the pen, Jody subtly reached over and placed her hand on my right leg. She pressed insistently, the third time in the meeting she had to deal with JiggleFoot.

We were buying our first house in a crazy Bay Area real estate market. Just to make the down payment, we had cleared out every bank account and borrowed money from parents. My pastor salary was going to be stretched mightily to afford the monthly payments looming before me like a life sentence. As we signed the documents, my face was calm and businesslike, but JiggleFoot gave me away. When I get nervous, I sit with my right leg crossed, and my right foot twitches rapidly and incessantly. JiggleFoot is Jody's Geiger counter for my anxious energy. The shakes per second indicate the intensity of the worries radiating out and bombarding her.

One of the most curious features of anxiety is just how much energy it generates and exhausts. Anxious energy can fuel physical activity such as pacing, hand-wringing, jitteriness, or other JiggleFoot-like activities. Rumination, worry, and discouragement can also consume our energy, disrupting our sleep and paralyzing our capacity to respond. In the same person, anxiety can sometimes alternate between generating and exhausting energy.

But here's the thing—regardless of the energy flow, the result overwhelmingly tends to be unproductive. JiggleFoot has been utterly useless in making a single mortgage payment. JiggleFoot has never accomplished anything other than unsettling Jody. The same could be said about pacing, rumination, obsession, and most other manifestations of anxious energy. Sometimes we find temporary ways to channel anxiety more usefully, but these momentary redirects rarely calm the underlying unrest fully. When I feel nervous, I will also obsessively tidy the house, but you can only rearrange the sofa cushions so many times. After arranging the cushions with a fastidiousness that would impress Martha Stewart, I finally sit down on the sofa, cross my legs, and give way to JiggleFoot. Want to experience the sheer power of anxious energy? Just try to stop JiggleFoot (or your unique version of it).

What is going on? Is there an opportunity to change our experience of anxious energy so we can lead more productive lives? If so, how?

Investigating Anxious Energy

A key biblical resource for investigating anxiety is the book of Psalms. Many of the prayers in the book contain some reference to emotional distress. The specific threats include the feared loss of one's reputation, physical security, financial provision, health, and more. The resulting symptoms are described as "worry," "fear," "terror," "hearts melting like wax," and unrelenting "sleep-lessness." Psalms is the prayer book for anxious people.

One especially important and famous prayer is Psalm 139. This particular prayer includes many of the themes already introduced in this book. For instance, the prayer issues an invitation to get present to God, the one who is always present to us such that the psalmist asks rhetorically, "Where can I flee from your presence?" (v. 7). This God recognizes the truths of our inner being, despite our attempts to deflect his searching presence, for, as the psalmist declares about God, "you know when I sit and when I rise; you perceive my thoughts from afar" (v. 2). What God sees in us, God accepts. He has embraced all of our multiple "selves": "For you created my inmost being; you knit me together in my mother's womb. I praise you because I am fearfully and wonderfully made; your works are wonderful, I know that full well" (vv. 13–14).

Psalm 139 culminates with an invitation to God to investigate the psalmist's anxiety: "Search me, God, and know my heart; test me and *know my anxious thoughts*" (v. 23, emphasis mine). In the ancient Hebrew worldview, "the heart" that is to be investigated represents the place of our deepest thinking. The ancient Hebrews did not have a conception of the brain like we moderns do, so they located the deepest flow of our thoughts—including our "anxious thoughts"—in the "heart."

If we do invite God to investigate our "anxious thoughts," what will happen? Psalm 139 informs us that God could locate some error in our anxious thoughts: "See if there is any offensive way in me, and lead me in the way everlasting" (v. 24).[1] Keep in mind that there is a difference between my feeling of anxiety and the error contained within me. Here is another reminder that the Bible never depicts the feeling of anxiety itself as a sin or moral offense. Anxiety is considered to be a normal and expected feature of life, and the psalmist assumes he will have "anxious thoughts." Yet those thoughts may contain an error that needs to be detected.

The purpose of this error detection is correction, not punishment or shame. God investigates our anxiety so that he can "lead me in the way everlasting." The end result is truly productive energy. God is leading us anew, and we are moving in a new way. And in that word *everlasting*, there is a renewable and sustainable quality to this energy.

The Anxiety Formula

In any investigation, a simple formula can make a big difference, especially when the phenomenon being examined is as complex as the nature of energy. Ideally, a formula simplifies complex realities to help us focus on the most important variables—the aspects we can change in order to achieve a desired result.

In 1905, a simple formula captured the fundamental nature of energy when Albert Einstein published his momentous $E = mc^2$ (Energy = mass × speed of light squared). This formula was built on complex calculations of elemental realities such as gravity, momentum, space, time and more. Most laypeople (including myself) cannot follow all of Einstein's underlying calculations, but $E = mc^2$ brilliantly synthesizes his many calculations into the relationship between the two most important variables—m (mass) and c, which is the notation for the speed of light.[2]

This synthesis into two variables enabled the average person to recognize the key insight—namely, that a huge amount of energy is contained in even a small amount of mass. C (the speed of light) is itself already a huge number; squaring c and multiplying it with mass produces *enormous* energy.

But in most cases, this energy is not readily available. E =

mc^2 tells us that huge amounts of energy are "trapped" within even a tiny piece of mass—like a pebble—but this trapped energy is usually in unusable form. The practical value of Einstein's formula was in focusing scientists on what to change. They knew that the speed of light is fixed, meaning it is impossible to change the c half of the equation. So the opportunity lay within the mass variable. Scientists eventually discovered that making small (subatomic, to be precise) changes in certain kinds of mass (radioactive elements in particular) could unlock enormous amounts of that trapped energy.[3] This approach resulted in world-changing applications, ranging from nuclear reactors to lasers to the Google Maps app on your phone.[4]

In our investigation of anxiety, we have now performed a variety of calculations on elemental realities of God, time, love, and death and described them through various Scriptures and stories. Now let's synthesize all these insights into something that can help us focus on what we can change to achieve practical results.

The Anxiety Formula is this:

Anxiety = Loss × Avoidance

According to this formula, the level of our anxiety is the product of two variables—loss and avoidance. Start with the first half of the equation:

Anxiety = **Loss** × Avoidance

Anxiety = Loss tells us that anxiety is generated by loss or, more specifically, by our fear of loss. Every anxiety is the fear of some future loss.

This is true of every type of anxiety. In health anxiety, we are hijacked into concerns about the future loss of bodily function. In financial anxiety, we fret about the future loss of money. In interpersonal anxiety, we fear the future loss of the regard of some person. In performance anxiety, we are concerned about the future loss of some aspect of our Ideal Self, such as being seen as competent or successful.

The Anxiety = Loss half of the equation reminds us once again that some level of anxiety is unavoidable. Anxiety is unavoidable because loss is unavoidable.

Why is loss unavoidable? Because it is the inescapable conclusion derived from calculating the most elemental realities of God, time, love, and especially death. Let's briefly summarize these calculations:

God: God is revealed most accurately in the person of Jesus. The gospel stories of Jesus confirm for us that God gets present with us in our anxiety, helps us recognize our anxiety, and lovingly accepts our anxious selves. But God does not prevent all loss *in our preresurrection lifetime*. The decisive evidence for this truth is that Jesus himself lost his life, showing that Christianity as a blueprint for avoiding loss during our lifetimes is simply false.

Time: Instead, God promises to restore all our losses in the final resurrection, the final feast. Until then, we live in the "Now and Not Yet" time. The time gap between the Now and the Not Yet inevitably exposes us to loss.

Love: We suffer anxiety because we are vulnerable to losing what we most love. This further explains why anxiety is unavoidable for anyone who is truly human. To be free of anxiety is to be free of any love (which is capable of being lost), which in turn would mean becoming inhuman. Sociopaths and psychopaths typically feel little anxiety because they feel little love and attachment to anything they might lose. But humans were made to love this world, with all of its experiences, things, values, and, above all, people. Anxiety thus can never be reduced to zero because to reduce the possibility of loss to zero is to reduce our humanity to zero. In the "Now and Not Yet" time, all human beings will lose their beloved objects.

Death: We all will lose our beloved objects because we are mortal human beings. We all will die. And in our death, we will lose every single beloved thing, experience, value, and person.

Pause for thirty seconds and ask yourself, *What do I most fear losing?* A job, an experience, the regard of another, a loved one? Bring that potential loss and fear to your mind. Do you have it?

Now think about this: *What is the likelihood I will suffer that particular loss at some point?* Try to assign a numerical percentage to that likelihood.

Whatever you chose, the correct answer is 100 percent. Whatever you love, you will lose. Because you will die. And when you die, you will lose every single thing, experience, value, and person you treasure.

For example, I fear losing productive activity. I'm one of those people who needs to be doing something useful all the time. Call me strange, but I'm worried about retirement. I can't imagine myself not working. I don't play golf or have any other all-consuming hobbies. In fact, hobbies have historically been hard for me to discover because I'm so wired for useful activity. Yet even if I never retire, I *will* lose productive activity in my life one day, because I *will* die one day. When that day comes, I will cease to be productive or useful. That loss—and all other losses—are guaranteed with 100 percent certainty.

This is anxiety's great and perverse irony. We experience anxiety as the uncertainty surrounding loss, but in actuality, all loss is absolutely certain. We can try to manage loss in our lives, like the probabilities of when a loss is likely to strike. But we quickly reach the limits of loss management. Death—like the speed of light—is fixed for all of us. It is unchanging. And the size of that loss is huge. In fact, it is total.

Keep in mind that *total* is not the same thing as *final*. Christianity does offer the hope that our loss will not be *final*. As we'll see later, properly grasping this *final* hope of resurrection is critical for our spiritual growth through anxiety. But many Christians can subconsciously believe that God is supposed to guarantee loss avoidance in life. Biblical Christianity never promises that we can avoid total loss in our lifetimes. Like Jesus, we all will die and experience the loss of everything. Like Jesus, we only access the final hope of resurrection by going through the total loss that awaits us all.

Therefore you're not being entirely delusional when you are anxious about loss. You are, in fact, facing an elemental truth. The delusion lies in believing we can ultimately avoid loss. Go back to the seemingly irrational chain of thought that triggered my panic attack by the pumpkin patch, where I ended up fearing the loss of my daughters, my wife, and my own life. I was being irrational in allowing myself to be so hijacked into the future that my body was responding to those losses as if they were actually happening to me at that moment. But I was not being irrational in realizing those losses at some point in the future. I will die, and when I do, I will lose my daughters, my wife, and my own life. To think I can avoid that loss is to delude myself into believing I can avoid the unavoidable.

The unavoidable reality of loss is why it is a fundamental mistake to treat anxiety itself as a problem we are supposed to eliminate. We can and should treat anxiety disorders, which stem from dysfunctional ways people respond to the experience of anxiety. But it is delusional to expect that we can or should eliminate anxiety itself. This delusion permeates Christians who treat anxiety as "sin."

It can also distort secular mental health approaches that treat anxiety as "disease." This was the point that social scientists Allan Horwitz and Jerome Wakefield made in their important book *All We Have to Fear*. They rightly call attention to various ways in which normal responses to the inevitable prospect of loss are increasingly pathologized by the mental health industry.[5]

To repeat, there is a critical difference between anxiety (which is inevitable) and anxiety disorders (which stem from dysfunctional responses to anxiety). And what is the most prevalent kind of dysfunctional response? It is *avoidance*.

This truth is captured in the second half of the Anxiety Formula:

Anxiety = Loss × Avoidance

Avoidance creates a multiplier effect. When we try to avoid the unavoidable, we are grabbing for something that will always be out of reach. That futile effort is the essence of anxious energy. The habits we adopt to avoid the unavoidable paradoxically increase anxiety. Avoidance is what charges the fixed reality of loss with the extra destructive energy we expend on worrying, fretting, and fearing. Our brains get trapped in futile loops, trying to do what is impossible. A leading scholar of the brain research on anxiety summarized the field's findings: "Excessive behavioral and/or cognitive avoidance is a leading hallmark of anxiety disorders."[6] Put in biblical terms, avoidance is at the core of that "offensive way" in our "anxious thoughts" described by Psalm 139:24.

Avoidance and Healing Prayer

Detecting avoidance—and the ways it multiplies anxiety—can be a tricky exercise. In fact, avoidance can be embedded in otherwise good and necessary spiritual practices, such as healing prayer.

Growing up as a Christian in a conservative evangelical church, I had little to no experience with healing prayer. When I arrived at Harvard as a freshman, I joined the Christian student fellowship on campus. I met and befriended Christians from more diverse backgrounds. For the first time, I got to know Black and Latino Pentecostals and other "charismatics" such as Whites from a church movement on the West Coast called the Vineyard. My new friends seemed to relate intensely with the Holy Spirit and talked often about their Spirit-filled experiences.

I grew spiritually from the example of my friends. I became more adventurous, even sort of "charismatic-adjacent." I dabbled at praying in tongues in worship and sought "words of knowledge." Understanding the Spirit's power and presence is indeed an enduring gift of the charismatic movement to the broader Christian church—and to me.

In the middle of my senior year, I suffered the biggest outbreak of anxiety I'd ever had in my life up to that point.

I woke up one morning with debilitating back pain. Since childhood, I've had congenital scoliosis (curvature of the spine) and even wore a bulky brace during part of my adolescent years. But the condition had never caused me serious pain. Until now. With one semester left to graduate, I could not sit in classes or work at a desk. I could not finish my senior honors thesis, which was a graduation requirement. I had to drop out of school. I was about to book my plane trip home to Chicago.

Uncertainty flooded my mind. *What if I never recover? Will this be the last time I'll see my friends?*

Anxiety hijacked me further into the future. I had envisioned going to graduate school and becoming a professor. In fact, I thought I had even received a "word of knowledge" that this was the future God intended for me. Suddenly it wasn't clear whether I'd ever get my undergraduate degree.

More potential losses piled up in my mind. *What if I become a permanent invalid? Will anyone find me attractive? Will I be able to get married? What about having kids?*

My Christian student fellowship was deeply important to me, so I postponed going home to Chicago and stayed with some friends off campus. The entire community rallied around me in prayer.

In one session, a friend brought up the idea of inviting a pastor who was known for his healing prayer ministry (who lived in another city) to come and pray for me. When the pastor agreed to do so, we felt this must be a sign that God was going to heal me.

In the days leading up to the arrival of this man, expectations within our close-knit fellowship grew. We had more intense times of prayer to prepare for the healing prayer session. Others began reporting words of knowledge from the Holy Spirit that something big would happen.

My friend who had invited the healer stopped by my room and leaned against the doorway. "I'm sure God is going to heal you somehow," he said.

"Really? Yeah, I guess I'm feeling excited too . . ." My voice trailed off a bit. "Uh, why are you feeling so confident?"

He was a logical kind of guy who was trained as a scientist. "I'm certain that God wants you to be part of our community, and you need to be healed to be here with us. Ergo, God is going to heal you."

Conflicting emotions and thoughts tossed within me. I desperately wanted him to be right. I wasn't sure I had received a definitive word of knowledge promising healing, but a surge of expectation swept through me. Something amazing surely was going to happen. Was this sense from God? Or from the excitement of my friends? Or from my own desperation? I did not know. But my friends were highly confident, and I was more than willing to be carried along.

Secretly, that Little Leaguer who feared being shamed and disappointing others was also present. I was afraid of what my community would think if the healing did not happen. This anxiety multiplied. *Do such fears mean I don't have faith? Could my lack of faith somehow block the healing? Or what if I were to commit a sin before the scheduled prayer session?* I started to worry I might look at some attractive girl on campus with lust in the hours before the session. I was afraid of screwing things up. I became even more scrupulous in scouring my conscience and confessing to God any hint of wrongdoing.

On the night of the prayer session, the pastor and a small group of my closest friends gathered around me in an off-campus apartment. The rest of the fellowship had gathered for a prayer vigil on campus. Some had been fasting in anticipation of this event.

The pastor was a kind and gentle older man. He laid hands on me and began to pray. The others joined in. There was prayer in tongues. People invoked the Holy Spirit. My friends "named and claimed" healing on my behalf.

And nothing happened.

I mean nothing happened in terms of a lasting physical healing. My back was not healed that night. Or since. I still have the same back condition to this day. Several weeks after that prayer session, I returned home to Chicago. I eventually learned to cope with the pain enough to return to school (and the Christian fellowship) the following year. I got my degree and went on with my life.

I also mean nothing happened in terms of how our fellowship made sense of this experience. For all the fervent prayer meetings, we never convened afterward to confront the reality that the Spirit did not come through in the way we expected. We avoided talking about the disappointment.

Our avoidance was understandable. Consider what we would've had to investigate. Was the lack of healing because those who claimed a "word of knowledge" were wrong? Or had I done something wrong? Those seemed like the two options on the table, but no one wanted to confront either of those possibilities. It would have been too uncomfortable for everyone. So we tried to forget about that particular experience and move on.

Except I couldn't. I had my expectations raised and then crushed—and that affected me. I'm not alone in having experienced this confusing deflation. Too many Christian communities (charismatic or otherwise) tend to avoid casting doubt on whether leaders heard God correctly in a promised healing, so the pressure of doubt backs up on the disappointed person.

Some who have experienced these kinds of dashed expectations end up doubting God (*maybe God doesn't exist*—or if God deliberately raised my hopes just to dash them, then *maybe God isn't that loving*). Others doubt themselves (*maybe I do lack faith* or *maybe I am harboring some hidden sin*). The confusion, doubts, and uncertainties are driven underground, but they are there. And left unaddressed, these spiritual anxieties can fester, multiply, and seep into our relationship with God.

Looking back, I now realize how that entire experience of healing prayer was charged throughout by the impulse to avoid loss. I wanted to avoid losing all my dreams for my future. My friends wanted to avoid losing my presence in the community. And when the healing didn't occur as expected, we all wanted to avoid losing spiritual confidence. All of this avoidance was understandable, well-meaning, and in fact filled with love. But the end result turned out to be greater levels of anxiety.

Let me be clear. I believe healing prayer is a good and necessary spiritual practice. I'm narrating my experience to illustrate how the impulse to avoid loss can lead a good practice astray, how it can become an "offensive way." Healing prayer can be practiced healthily—without the spiritual distortion caused by our need to avoid loss, without overstating our level of certainty, without the need to assign blame for unanswered prayers. But when our avoidance impulse goes unrecognized, we can easily slip into more damaging forms of healing prayer and end up multiplying our anxiety.

Avoidance Habits

Spiritual avoidance multiplies spiritual anxiety. This happens with bad habits such as "name it and claim it" and "pray anxiety away." Those spiritual habits push away the possibility of loss, which creates more spiritual anxiety: *Maybe I don't have enough faith. . . . Maybe I have a hidden sin. . . . Maybe God doesn't love me. . . . Maybe God is a sadist.*

Physical avoidance multiplies physical anxiety. With physical-related phobias such as claustrophobia, the sufferer wishes to avoid placing their body into constrained spaces. This requires focusing on the constraining aspects of all spaces. Over time, the body becomes hypersensitized to how close walls and ceilings are everywhere. As physical avoidance becomes more ingrained in habits, this sensitivity grows such that even the smallest hint of constraint can generate intense physical symptoms of panic.[7]

Mental avoidance multiplies mental anxiety. Think back with me to my latchkey kid days. If I could find out my mom's exact departure, I'd fend off my fears. Right? Wrong. One snowstorm in a Chicago winter (as inevitable as death itself) catapulted my fear level. Knowing her precise departure and expected arrival—data intended to avoid uncertainty—ironically magnified each turn of the clock's minute hand, driving up my worries by the second.

As was true in my healing prayer experience, avoidance habits can be subtle. Take the anxious parent. Some parents cross over from appropriate levels of attention into helicoptering. It may seem like helicopter parents are practicing the opposite of avoidance. But helicoptering is charged with anxious avoidance. Helicopter parents desperately try to avoid facing the inevitability that their children will suffer loss. They are deluding themselves that "we can fix everything" in order to prevent loss. This underlying avoidance contaminates what otherwise can be healthy parental attention.

Other parents may veer from appropriately giving their kids room to becoming disengaged. A disengaged parent seems like the opposite of a helicopter parent. But if you dig beneath the surface, you'll often find anxiety and avoidance. Disengaged parents usually are threatened by their children's inevitable suffering (as well as by the loss of their own self-image as a competent parent). They tell themselves "everything is fine." That underlying avoidance contaminates what otherwise can be a healthy space for kids to grow. "We can fix everything" and "everything is fine" both grow out of anxiety; they're just different avoidance habits.

When we drill underneath the many seemingly opposite surface reactions, we find this shared connection. The stressed-out student and the lazy slacker are both fueled by a desire to avoid failure (which is a loss of some aspect of their Ideal Self). The former avoids by overworking, while the latter avoids by not trying. Think of the hypochondriac and the person who refuses to get a checkup. The former avoids the inevitability of death by turning over every single diagnostic card, the latter by refusing to turn over any.

This makes sense because anxiety hijacks the fight-or-flight system designed by God. To avoid an immediate threat, we are hardwired to mobilize our energy to either circle *around* (fight) or back *away* (flight) from the threat. The helicoptering parent, stressed-out student, and hypochondriac circle *around* the fear (in order to avoid loss). The disengaged parent, slacker student, and checkup refuser veer *away* from the fear (also to avoid loss). Both sides are avoiding the prospect of loss with different habits. Identifying our own particular avoidance habit—whether *around* or *away*—can provide a practical insight. It tells us which countermeasures we need to take to lower our anxiety.[8]

Regardless of which type of avoidance habit is in play, the result is anxious energy. Avoidance generates anxious energy because we are trying to avoid the unavoidable. It only produces futility. Because we're attempting to achieve the impossible, ever more energy must be summoned to keep our avoidance move going. This is why anxiety feels simulta-

> **Trying to avoid the unavoidable generates anxious energy.**

neously exhausting and addictive. The anxious person is trapped on the proverbial hamster wheel. The faster they run—either *around* or *away* from their fears—the more they get nowhere. Avoidance habits trap anxious energy.

The Opportunity for Change

The Anxiety Formula shows us that *lowering avoidance is a powerful way to lower anxiety.*

Like $E = mc^2$, Anxiety = Loss × Avoidance identifies the

opportunity for change. Avoidance is the key variable. Like the speed of light, loss is fixed, inevitable, and huge (in fact, total) over the course of our lifetimes. But just as subatomic changes in mass can greatly affect energy levels, modest changes in lowering avoidance can greatly affect anxiety levels. In the process, anxious energy can get freed up into more productive energy. Unlocking this opportunity requires changing how we handle avoidance.

We can change our avoidance habits. A large body of psychological research shows that lowering avoidance can meaningfully lower anxiety.[9] But lowering avoidance requires *training*. Avoidance habits are deeply ingrained in us, often starting early in our childhood (like my latchkey kid ploy). Through repetition, they become unconscious and habitual. Thus, lowering avoidance habits requires practice.

Avoidance habits also call us to undertake a deeper investigation. In some cases, our avoidance is charged with a dark spiritual energy. We sometimes have to drill to this nuclear core, which the Bible calls "idolatry." Indeed, some versions of Psalm 139 conclude the process of inviting God to "investigate our anxious thoughts," with verse 24 translated as, "Look to see if there is any *idolatrous* way in me" (CEB, emphasis added). An idol is anything that supplants the rightful role of God—especially his love for us—in our lives. Idolatry is the set of habits that embodies our trust in this alternative to God's love. In some cases, idolatry pulsates at the center of anxiety because idolatry is all about avoidance—avoiding our need to trust God.

Let me emphasize that idolatry is not always at the core of every case of anxiety, only that it could be. This is why the writer of Psalm 139 invites God to search his anxious thoughts to see if there is "any idolatrous way" in him. And the discovery of idolatry at the nuclear core of one's anxiety is actually an incredible opportunity: if one can smash that idol, it is like the spiritual equivalent of smashing the atom. Incredible amounts of trapped energy can be freed up for the kind of productivity God intends for us.

How do we apply this Anxiety Formula to our lives in a practical manner? How do we lower our avoidance such that anxiety is lowered and anxious energy is transformed into productive and renewable energy, into what Psalm 139 describes as "the way everlasting"? How do we identify hidden idolatry that might lie at the core of a particular anxiety? The next chapter provides a case study in using the Anxiety Formula.

CHAPTER 9

What Do You Have to Lose?

Whang! Whang! Whang!

The claxon-sounding alarm startled me out of my office chair. It was Monday, March 16, 2020.

I swiveled, trying to locate the source of this unfamiliar sound and finally realized it was blaring from the phone in my pocket. I pulled it out to read the announcement. My county was declaring a stay-at-home order, effective that day.

Santa Clara County—like others in the Bay Area—was among the first to implement a lockdown in response to what was the hazily recognized threat of COVID-19. The Bay Area locked down faster and more drastically than practically every other region in the country.

Later, I went to the grocery store for supplies. The streets were already thinning out, acquiring the feeling of a ghost town. At the store, however, a long line had formed, and some shelves were completely empty.

Over the next weeks, the virus and uncertainty spread. My anxiety climbed so fast I was throwing all my practices at it. For instance, I went on repeated bike rides to try to get present via nature. It looked like I was hopping on my bike, but really I was hopping on the back of my anxious thoughts and getting carried away into anxiety's scary scenarios of the future. *What's going to happen next? How long is this lockdown going to last? Is everything going to fall apart?* I returned from those rides more worried than I was when I started out.

Part of me was tempted to deflect my attention to issues "out there." I told myself my real problem was a lack of data about what was happening in the world. I obsessively scanned the internet for the latest case counts, research findings, and reports from far-away places such as Wuhan and Italy. Somewhere in my Google search history is the phrase "Tom Hanks blood oxygen levels."

Despite this deflection to "out there," I began to recognize anxiety was "in here." In fact, I could precisely measure its rise within my body. Because of my recently diagnosed heart defect (which also made me more vulnerable to the threat of COVID-19), I wear a heart rate monitor on my bike rides. Normally, as I pedal, I can see my rate climb steadily from white to blue to green (the target training rate), and I take care to keep it below yellow and definitely below red. On one of those rides in the early days of the lockdown, I was startled to see I was starting out already in green. Even modest exertion took me into yellow and even red.

I was still such an anxious person that I couldn't even exercise normally. I started to berate myself for not being more mature, for not having achieved as much spiritual progress as I thought I had. Summoning my "acceptance move" was especially important in those moments. When I recognized my self-hatred kicking in, I reached over with my right hand and gently patted my left shoulder. I kept telling myself, *It's all right, kiddo. It's all right.*

Going through these and other practices helped slow my rise in anxiety. And throughout this time, I prayed regularly, engaging especially in my contemplative prayer practice. However, while the climb of anxiety slowed, it did not stop. Three weeks into the lockdown, I recognized that my sleep was deteriorating. A sobering warning sign.

Moreover, in my prayer times, the Holy Spirit stirred in me. This was a kind of unease, but different in quality from anxiety's unease. It was a "holy unease," which didn't trap me in my own looping thoughts; it felt instead like an invitation, a call to action.

The public health world was furiously researching the medical nature of the pandemic. I realized that the Spirit was calling me to investigate the spiritual nature of my anxiety.

Where to start?

Dig into Loss

The Anxiety Formula (Anxiety = Loss × Avoidance) tells us to start by trying to identify the precise nature of the feared loss because lowering our avoidance habits in that space will have the most outsized impact. This takes effort because we naturally avoid going there. We tend to bury awareness of our more feared losses deeply in our psyches, often underneath other lesser losses. We need to dig.

When I first started to investigate my pandemic anxiety, I assumed I was most worried about my health, especially given my recent heart diagnosis. I engaged in my mental radio practice, where I deliberately listen—with the Spirit of Jesus alongside—to my anxious thoughts from a differentiated posture. I discovered a surprise: KFEAR wasn't nearly as loud as KWORK. My thoughts were mostly about my consulting firm. And KWORK had apparently been acquired by KFEAR in a hostile corporate takeover.

In the pandemic, this new KFEAR was getting louder . . . and edgier, like it had become an urban rap station. If my looping thoughts could be rendered as an amateur rap song, the lyrics would sound something like this:

> *Pan-demic is eco-nomic*
> *A lockdown be a meltdown*
> *Funding cuts trendin'*
> *Nonprofits non spendin'*
> *My clients go away*
> *So who gonna pay?*
>
> *I say and I say*
> *Every effin' day:*
> *Who gonna pay?*
> *Who gonna pay?*

I know what you're saying: "Curtis, if you're thinking of becoming a rap artist, well, uh . . . don't quit your day job." But that was the point. What if I *was* forced to quit my day job?

Who gonna pay? I had already led my firm through the 2008–2009 Great Recession. I knew that in a severe and prolonged economic downturn, nonprofit spending on consulting services like mine was the first to get cut and the last to come back. In the spring of 2020, many experts were predicting an even more severe and prolonged economic collapse. Was my firm going to survive this one? My fear of losing my company was underneath my anxiety, and the Spirit was taking me there.

How to Recognize the Voice of the Spirit

We are all invited to "go there," for this kind of mental digging into our feared losses can be practiced by anyone. But the need to investigate our own thoughts prompts a helpful detour from our pandemic story into an important methodological question: How do Christians recognize the voice of the Holy Spirit? How do we know we're hearing from someone other than ourselves?

The question is one about the origin of *thoughts* in particular because most Christians do not hear the Holy Spirit audibly. KFEAR—and the insights generated from listening to it—were not playing from an external speaker, but rather in my thoughts. When investigating your fears, thoughts arise in your head from any number of inner sources. It is difficult to establish whether what you're hearing is originating from the Spirit or from yourself.

This difficulty in separating out the Spirit from our self can paralyze Christians when it comes to investigating our own thoughts. One way some Christians try to resolve this challenge is by prizing insights that could have *only* originated from the voice of the Spirit *alone*. In some charismatic communities, this means an especially intense desire for "words of knowledge," where they believe God delivered divine information to recipients from an outside source (like another person) in a way that was purely external, such that there can be no possibility that the information originated from within one's own self. In these settings, you will hear people validate a word of knowledge by claiming, "There was no way he could have known that!"

I believe that the Spirit does sometimes speak via a word of knowledge from the outside and in ways that preclude any source internal to one's own mind. The Bible certainly includes examples of this miraculous dynamic. However, the basic nature of the Spirit should encourage us not to demand this kind of sharp separation between the Spirit's voice and our own inner thoughts.

The biblical understanding of the Holy Spirit moves us away from a sharp "either-or" distinction, where we split our thoughts from the Spirit's voice. Romans 8:26 describes the Holy Spirit as the Searcher of Hearts. Remember, in the ancient Jewish taxonomy, the heart was the home of deep thoughts. So the Holy Spirit's role is to investigate our thoughts. The same verse emphasizes that this Searcher comes *alongside* us—not as an external speaker who is distant from us.

Jesus describes our connection with the Holy Spirit in even more intimate and internal terms. In extended passages like John 14–17, Jesus repeatedly locates the Spirit as living *within us*, as one who will "guide you into all the truth" (John 16:13). This means the Spirit within us will guide us into all the truth already within us, regardless of its previous origin. We should expect that the Searcher of Hearts will search for usable raw material in our existing thoughts to co-fashion new insights. Our relationship with the Spirit is not "either-or." The question "Does this thought originate *either* from the Spirit *or* from me?" is the wrong question.

When digging through our thoughts, the right evaluative question is "Does this thought sound like Jesus in tone and content?"

Consider listening to the voice of the Spirit as a practice of seeking vocal fidelity. In the field of acoustics, "vocal fidelity" refers to how closely an audio sample matches the original source. Applied to the spiritual field, the principle of vocal fidelity is based on the truth that the Holy Spirit is the spirit of Jesus, and Jesus promises that his Spirit will take what is his and make it known to us (John 16:14). The Spirit will only guide us in ways faithful to the way Jesus would guide us.

This is why reading the Gospels is so important for Christians, specifically for those who seek to hear the voice of the Spirit. Reading the Gospels (especially in such a way that we are placed in the narrative) is like listening to the "master recording." As we read about Jesus, we develop our voice recognition skills. We grow in discerning which of our inner thoughts bear "vocal fidelity" to the Master. This kind of inner spiritual

117

growth is much more fruitful and reliable than our desperate need to receive an external "word of knowledge" whenever we experience anxiety. In fact, investigating our anxious thoughts is a wonderful growth opportunity to practice our ability to hear the Spirit through the application of the principle of "vocal fidelity."

Spirit-voiced insights are those that bear *tonal fidelity* to Jesus. If we hear accusatory, shaming, fearful, or anxious voices, these words most likely do not originate from the Spirit. They are the words of some other inner voices projecting themselves. We know this because Jesus does not sound accusatory, shaming, fearful, or anxious in the Gospels.

An insight that originates from the Spirit will also bear *theological fidelity* to Jesus in its content. If we think we've heard the Spirit promising to save us from a specific loss with absolute certainty, this could be our avoidance impulse projecting because Jesus, in contrast to our impulses, spends much more time teaching his disciples the certainty that they should expect to lose all things (e.g., Matthew 16:24–26; Luke 18:24–34).

When digging into our feared loss, the principle of vocal fidelity makes it much more likely that what we will hear from the Spirit will take the form of a question. A skillful question—much more than a pronounced conclusion—is how Jesus co-fashioned insights with his students. Jesus was continually asking questions. Biblical scholar Martin Copenhaver showed that Jesus asked question after question (in fact, 307 of them in the Gospels). This method of co-fashioning truth far surpassed how often he answered questions with declarative statements.[1] Question asking is how the Spirit of Jesus frequently comes alongside us to guide us—and not force us—toward the truth.

What we hear from the Spirit will likely take the form of a question.

When it comes to anxiety, we should especially be alert to the "why" questions that come from the Spirit. "*Why* are you afraid?" was the question Jesus asked the anxious disciples in the middle of the storm (Mark 4:35–41) and to a worried Mary Magdalene outside the empty tomb (John 20:13).

Let's now apply these spiritual insights about how the Spirit speaks back to my pandemic story. Listening to KFEAR told me I was worried about losing my consulting firm. But the Spirit gently kept coming alongside and digging within my thoughts: *Why exactly do I fear this so much?*

In one of my contemplative prayer times, an answer crystallized in my mind: COVID-19 was threatening my Ideal Self. My company represented a way the world now looked at me—as a successful entrepreneur. After my failure as a pastor, I had worked hard to develop this new identity. Losing my company would mean losing that part of my Ideal Self.

Digging to this next layer of loss helped me identify the associated avoidance move I could change. My Ideal Self tries to avoid losing the admiration of others by banishing the Anxious Self from public view. Because the Anxious Self is unavoidably part of me, this avoidance move backfires and leads to more anxiety. Lowering anxiety thus meant lowering this particular avoidance move. I needed to stop banishing my Anxious Self from public view. How could I do this?

My response was to email some of my Christian friends around the country—deliberately including those to whom I wanted to present only my Ideal Self. In the email, I shared my fear about losing my company and asked for their prayers. Many of them responded with sympathy, intercession, and acceptance. Their kindness helped me accept my Anxious Self and reconcile it with my Ideal Self.

Everyone has their own particular layers of loss. While the

loss of some aspect of the Ideal Self is present for many, you may find some other kind of loss underneath your mental surface. The Anxiety = Loss formula only tells you to dig into your feared losses; it doesn't tell you how the layers are arranged. The only way to know for yourself is to pray the prayer of Psalm 139 and ask God to search *you* and know *your* anxious thoughts. The Spirit of God is a personal guide, not a formula. If you are open, the Searcher of Hearts will dig along with and within you. If you listen for the voice of the Master, you may hear the question gently posed: *Why? Why does this loss feel so fearful?*

Reach the Limits of Loss Management

Digging to the deeper layers of the Loss part of the Anxiety Formula also equips us to reach the limits of loss management. Even though we cannot ever absolutely avoid Loss, we can sometimes manage its edges. For instance, I will lose my physical life eventually. Nevertheless, I still exercise regularly to tilt the odds that this loss will happen later. I also exercise so that in the time I have remaining, I can be maximally active and productive.

Engaging in practical steps of loss management can help reduce some anxiety. Doing productive tasks is better than being paralyzed with worry. Work can help distract us from looping thoughts. Exercise releases stress-alleviating hormones.

However, all of that is simply loss management, not loss avoidance. I cannot ever exercise enough to avoid death—the Loss of all losses. To remind ourselves of the limits of loss management, my wife and I have hung a sign over the barbells in our home workout space that reads "This Mortal Coil Gym"—and it is painted in black with a drawing of a skull. It is a small literary joke—a reference to Hamlet's soliloquy about the inevitability of death ("when we have shuffled off this mortal coil")—but it is also meant to be a serious reminder of our limits in loss management.

When it comes to spiritual growth, it is crucial to recognize the limits of our management steps. As I dealt with my feared loss of my company, I focused on managing the odds during those early months of the pandemic. I stayed close to my customers, diversified my service offerings, and carefully watched my cash flow. *None of these steps promise certainty*, I reminded myself. These reminders especially helped keep me from overworking beyond healthy limits, especially during a crisis. We're tempted to overwork most when we mistakenly believe the completion of that next task is what will decisively rescue us from uncertainty—and thus we can't stop working.

Even as I tried to save my company in the pandemic, I tried to remind myself of the parable of the rich fool (Luke 12:16–21), where the man seeks to manage potential loss by building up ever more savings in bigger barns—only to have God say, "You fool! This very night your life will be demanded from you. Then who will get what you have prepared for yourself?" In this and other parables, Jesus is warning us that we can grossly exaggerate our ability to manage loss with any certainty. This is true of every loss management move. It happens all the time—people who eat right and exercise regularly still end up receiving an unexpected diagnosis of terminal illness.

In my loss management steps, I also prayed for practical help. I asked God to provide concrete answers to the worrisome question of *Who gonna pay?* I prayed for more paying clients. The Bible encourages us to ask God for whatever we need (see Luke 18:1–8). But in asking God to support our loss management efforts, we must not overreach. There is an important line between request and presumption, between hope and certainty.

Remember that all our prayers to God in the Now and Not

Yet are affected by uncertainty. Soon after I emailed my friends for prayer support, one particularly lucrative project arose. Because of the timing, I assumed God was surely answering my prayers. But at the last second, the project fell through. On the other hand, other projects fell into my lap even after a long time had elapsed since my last prayer request. Why?

Why this unpredictability? Is this God's way of limiting our temptation to relate to him as consumers, treating him impersonally like a Cosmic Amazon that delivers everything we think we need with one prayer click?

We are meant to relate to God as his children. Our Father God's gift giving is more personal, more like my mom's gift giving at Christmas. Sometimes she gives me exactly what I need, with prescience (like when I didn't realize my old wallet was wearing out until she gave me a new one); other times, she gives me a head scratcher (*Mom, you know I don't like scarves!*). Her unpredictability is part of the reality that she is a person. She is a parent with her own ideas (*and who knows, maybe the secret of good health is indeed maintaining consistent neck temperature!*), not a service at my mechanistic command. Perhaps God's unpredictability is an expression of his personhood and parenthood.

This is a theory. I don't really know for sure why our Father God supports some of our loss management steps and not others. I will receive my answer when the gap between the Now and the Not Yet finally closes. Until then, I remain uncertain.

During the pandemic, reaching and respecting the limits of loss management did bring some relief to several anxiety symptoms. My sleep stabilized, and I was able to return to exercising at a normal heart rate. But my rumination annoyingly persisted. I needed to keep investigating this particular form of anxious energy.

The Spirit had been co-investigating with me my feared loss. It was time to turn to the second half of the Anxiety Formula.

CHAPTER 10

How We Try to Avoid Loss

The second half of the Anxiety Formula (Anxiety = Loss x Avoidance) points us to the variable that most significantly determines our anxiety levels—our avoidance. While we should dig into and identify the loss we fear, we will eventually reach the limits of loss management. In many specific situations, we cannot do much to change the actual quantity of imminent loss; most importantly, when considering our lives in whole, we are utterly helpless. Total loss—death itself—awaits us all.

Therefore, the quantity of anxiety over the whole course of our lives will be determined by our quantity of avoidance. We *can* change things here. To do so, we have to first identify how avoidance has become habitual. In this chapter, I want to explain the nature of avoidance habits and illustrate them along the way with examples from my pandemic story.

Identify Avoidance Habits

My most persistent expression of anxiety during the pandemic took the form of rumination. Rumination is an example of an *around* avoidance habit. Like a helicopter parent hovering around one's children, my thoughts were looping around my company in a futile attempt to avoid the loss. My mind was still somehow trapped in the "I can fix everything" delusion. Recall that other people avoid loss with *away* avoidance habits, where their thoughts veer away from a topic in an equally futile attempt to avoid the loss. Their minds are like the disengaged parent, telling themselves "everything is fine."

To decrease avoidance, it is helpful to identify your particular avoidance habit. You need to know what habit is trapping you in order to take the right countermeasures.

Here are some common habits, some of which may be familiar to you.

Away (Flight) Habits	Around (Fight) Habits
Avoiding certain conversations	Rumination (looping thoughts)
Social media addiction	Obsessive-compulsive behavior
Shopping impulses	Rehearsing scenarios (past or present)
Workaholism and/or compulsive busyness	Badgering others
Addiction to alcohol, drugs, or pornography	Inability to let go

Of course, any one person can practice avoidance habits from both sides of the chart. But in my experience, people gravitate toward one side or the other, consistent with whether they tend to be "flight" or "fight" people. Generally speaking, I'm a fight guy, and my rumination is the mental expression of my fight tendency.

Think of these two types of avoidance habits as handling two different types of balls—a rubber ball or a ball of dough.

Away habits are like handling one of those bouncy, rubber

"super balls." If you can imagine your feared loss as one of those balls, *away* moves are like throwing the ball away from you but then having it bounce back in your face.

There are some classic examples of *away* habits. For instance, people often avoid talking about a subject matter that raises the possibility of loss. Some people avoid talking about money or diseases because they fear financial or health loss. Underneath social media addiction, especially for teens, is the desire to avoid the loss of some connection with peers. Society has even coined a name for that fear—FOMO (Fear of Missing Out). For many adults (and teens), social media is a way to distract themselves from the fear of solitude or emptiness.

Notice how many of these *away* habits can escalate into addictions of various sorts. *Away* habits are highly addictive because each one provides a temporary reprieve from the possibility of loss. But these habits cannot make that real possibility disappear. So we have to keep going back for another hit.

In fact, whenever we're pushing something unavoidable *away*, it will bounce back with greater force. So we have to engage in higher levels of away habits to push it away again—only to see it bounce back with greater energy. And so on and so on and so on.

That bounce back is the essence of addiction. This is why most substance abuse treatments have an anxiety treatment component. So much of substance abuse is trying to distract or numb away loss, especially the possibility of more loss in the future.

In comparison, an *around* habit is like handling a ball of dough. If you imagine your feared loss in this way, an *around* habit is turning that loss around and around—as the ball gets progressively stickier.

Around habits are especially tricky to identify as avoidance because it seems like we're doing the opposite of avoidance. It seems like we're facing the loss and heading toward the threat. That's part of the deceptive trick. *Around* habits make it appear like we're dealing with the issue of loss because we're constantly thinking, repeating behavior, rehearsing mentally, or badgering others around the possibility of loss. But we're still practicing avoidance. It is true that we're not avoiding the subject matter itself, but at the deepest level, we're still trying to avoid the loss.

Whereas *away* habits bounce back with greater force, *around* habits get more and more sticky. Anxiety has tricked you into thinking, *If I turn it over one more time, if I can look at this from every possible angle, if I can cover every base, then the possibility of loss will go away.* But the final turn, the final angle, the final base *does not exist*. The possibility of loss is always still there. So if my mind keeps going around and around the situation, trying to avoid any possibility of loss, I won't be able to let go of the anxiety. It will grip me. I will get more and more anxious.

Identifying our specific avoidance habits—and their futile and addictive nature—prepares us to make changes to lessen our addiction. We will be truly motivated to stop an addictive behavior only when we realize the behavior is getting us nowhere and we're wasting our energy. With my pandemic-triggered rumination about my company's prospects, I finally started to recognize it for what it truly was—a sticky ball of dough I was turning around and around in my hands. Having that picture in my mind strengthened my resolve to stop.

Breaking Addiction to Avoidance Habits

Avoidance habits, like any addiction, become ingrained in our minds. Neuroscience has shown actual physical ingraining happens constantly in our brains. Any action establishes a neural pathway in our brain; repeated actions deepen that pathway.

Addictions are like destructive pathways where the grooves have gotten etched deeply over time, and we become mired in those ruts.

A key to breaking any addiction is *stopping* that etching process as much as we can and *replacing* it with new actions that lay alternative—and healthier—neural pathways. This "stop and replace" work rarely happens suddenly, which is why the practical goal is to decrease (versus immediately eliminate) avoidance habits over time.

My avoidance habit was rumination, an invisible mental action. I found it helpful to make the "stop and replace" work more visible and physical. The more senses we engage, the more neural pathways we can affect. My daughter made me a small wooden box, which I placed on my bedside table. I call it my "God Box." When I recognize I'm trapped in a rumination, I write it out on a slip of paper and place it in the "God Box" and ask the Spirit to help me close that box and keep it shut. Whenever I found myself ruminating about my company, I pictured myself as a slightly mischievous child caught with his hand in the cookie jar. I then imagined the Spirit gently but firmly asking me to put the unhealthy thought back in the box.

Note how the replacement practice for my *around* addiction has an *away* quality to it. I was quite physically putting the thought away. Engaging in this kind of countermeasure leverages the natural energy in our fight-or-flight system to break addictions. This is why it is helpful to identify our avoidance habits as landing in one side or the other of the *around* versus *away* divide. This identification gives some clue as to practices that can counterbalance our addiction. These countermeasures (as long as they don't become addictive themselves) can help replace the neural pathways of the addictive practice with new neural pathways.

For people stuck in *away* pathways, it may be helpful to

consider actions that take their minds *around* the feared loss in some manageable doses. Psychologists call this countermeasure "exposure therapy."[1] If you are addicted to *away* habits, consider how you can expose yourself to limited and controlled doses of feared loss. If you use my "God Box" idea, you can write out the underlying loss being avoided and deposit that slip of paper into the box. Whenever you are tempted to engage in an *away* habit to stave off loss (like social media consumption), take out that slip of paper and prayerfully contemplate that loss for ten minutes. This will expose you to the possible loss and may lessen its grip on you.

I am generally not an *away* guy, but I do have personal experience with addiction to one version of *away* habits. Several years ago, I was spending more and more of my evenings surfing the internet to research purchases for things I didn't need. In fact, I was inventing needs to feed my habit. (*Jody, don't we need an electric pepper grinder? No? How about an air fryer?*) I didn't crave the object itself (*Well, okay, I did want the air fryer*); what I craved was the neurological hit of doing the research. Whenever I was bored, I wanted that hit. Why did I need to run away from even the hint of boredom?

There were clues. First, this addiction started ramping up as I neared my fiftieth birthday. Second, I experienced this urge in the evenings after I had stopped working. For years, evenings were filled with parenting duties, whether putting the kids to bed when they were much younger or helping them with homework as they got older. But at this point, they didn't need or want any of my help.

I realized that the loss I was fearing was the loss of productive activity. Researching the best electric pepper grinder gave me a momentary sensation of usefulness. (*Jody, come on, think of the massive gains in productivity from not having to grind pepper by hand!*) It was an *away* move, fleeing from my underlying fear of not having anything to do.

In this case, my countermeasure was to lean in the *around* direction. This is where my existing practice of contemplative prayer was helpful. Contemplative prayer is like a spiritual "exposure therapy" where we're exposed to the loss of usefulness. It is meeting God while surrounded by silence and stillness. In contemplative prayer, nothing we do has any purpose other than being in that space. So whenever I recognized a sensation of boredom and a corresponding urge to research potential purchases to give me something to do, I tried to engage in twenty minutes of contemplative prayer. At first, it was hard to stay in that posture for that long, as I felt restless to get away from this sensation of lacking purpose. But the more I let stillness flow all around me, the more I could tolerate not having anything to do. Over time, this countermeasure significantly lowered my addiction.

To break your own addictions, you will need to find your own countermeasure. The best ones will be the ones you co-fashion with the Spirit. Ask the Spirit for guidance and listen for ideas that bear "vocal fidelity" to Jesus.

As you do, listen especially for the tonal qualities of patience and grace. Lessening addiction takes time, and you'll usually experience a "three steps forward, two steps back" feel to the process. Remember the promise of Romans 8:26: The Spirit comes alongside and "helps us in our weakness."

Repent of Underlying Idolatry

Let's clarify one more time the relationship between anxiety and sin. Anxiety itself is not sin. It is an inevitable part of what it means to be humans living in the Now and Not Yet. And most avoidance habits—as dysfunctional as they are—are more accurately understood as "bad habits" than as outright sin. However, it is possible in some cases that the sin of idolatry can be lurking underneath anxious thoughts. This is precisely why the author of Psalm 139 asks God to "search my anxious thoughts" in order to ascertain if there is "any idolatrous way in me" (CEB).

As we dig deeper into our feared losses, we may uncover the particular sin of idolatry. Remember our earlier definition of idolatry? Idolatry is avoidance directed at God, where we are avoiding having to trust in his love and provision for us.

We need to examine anxiety for the presence of underlying idolatry because idols rely on anxiety to gain allegiance from humans. An idol preys on our human vulnerability to uncertainty. It promises avoidance of uncertainty and loss in order to woo people away from God.

Take the scene from Isaiah 40–41. The chapters open with God reassuring Israel of his love, even though he is taking them through an intensely anxious moment in world history. The Assyrian Empire is sweeping through the nations of the ancient Near East. God's words to the Israelites are like a loving mother's reassurance to an anxious child: "Comfort, comfort my people, says your God. Speak tenderly to Jerusalem" (40:1–2).

However, God's loving comfort is not to be equated with a promise that Israel will avoid the loss of their land, their independence, their political status, and other treasured things. God is using the Assyrian invasion to correct the nations, including Israel. Meaningful losses will occur. God invites his people to trust him *through* those losses and not try to *avoid* them.

But the people of God want avoidance. So they turn to metalworkers and goldsmiths to make an idol to supplant Israel's God as the one who cares for them (Isaiah 40:18–20).

Isaiah 41:5–7 depicts how they promote allegiance to the idol:

The islands have seen it and fear;
    the ends of the earth tremble.
They approach and come forward;
    they help each other
    and say to their companions, "Be strong!"
The metalworker encourages the goldsmith,
    and the one who smooths with the hammer
    spurs on the one who strikes the anvil,
One says of the welding, "It is good."
    The other nails down the idol so it will not
        topple.

The idol promises that uncertainty and loss can be avoided, with the physical stability of the idol itself ("so it will not topple") meant to represent the promised political, social, and military certainty. To reiterate, the passage is not saying anxiety itself is idolatry. The sin is not in the "islands" being filled with "fear" or "the ends of the earth" being prone to "tremble." The sin is in believing the idol can provide a way to avoid those anxieties. The ensuing idol-making constructs an alternative to the loving comfort offered by God in Isaiah 40:1–2. This is why the idol makers of 41:5–7 are depicted as grunting to each other a farcical version of God's reassurance and tenderness: "Be strong!" and "It is good." Indeed, their words sound like the thin reassurances often offered to anxious people today such as, "Don't worry; it will all work out."

In the ancient world, idolatry preyed on human anxiety by making false promises of certainty. This is why idols proliferated wherever uncertainty was present. There was an idol to sacrifice to before the unknowns of a long journey; another idol to pray to when a child got sick; yet another idol with whom to share a meal at the onset of the unpredictable harvest, and so on and so on. Idols intertwine themselves with our basic human impulse to avoid loss.

How do we discern when our avoidance habits are wrapped in an underlying idolatry? How do we locate the dark nuclear core?

Once again, we need the Holy Spirit's active partnership in the spiritual investigation of our anxiety. The Anxiety Formula only tells us where idolatry (if present) is most likely hiding— intertwined with our deepest losses and most addictive avoidance habits. It doesn't predict that idolatry is always present or give us the precise identity of that idol. The same avoidance habit in different people can have a different spiritual diagnosis. One person's rumination could be just that—a bad mental habit that needs to be lessened gradually; another's could be charged by a subtle idolatry calling for repentance now.

The Spirit makes fine and critical distinctions in "the thoughts and attitudes of the heart" (Hebrews 4:12). The Searcher of Hearts helps us detect the presence of sin in our inner thoughts (John 16:8). Ultimately, to discern the presence of idolatry within our avoidance habits, each of us needs to practice hearing this voice.

While I can't offer a formula that will give you the precise coordinates and identity of your idol (if one indeed exists under-neath your anxieties), I can provide one more tip on how to listen: *pay attention to your defensiveness.*

In those anxious days of the pandemic as I progressed through my investigative steps, a curious new resistance to fur-ther digging arose in me. I usually welcome self-examination, so this was strange. In particular, I noticed I was resisting further spiritual questioning along these lines: "Why were my mental *around* habits still orbiting furiously around my company in particular?" As mentioned, I had initially discerned that the feared loss of my company was about the loss of my Ideal Self as a successful entrepreneur, and I thought that this revelation would settle the investigation. But the Spirit kept prodding me with more questions about why I was still ruminating about my company.

Our emotional reaction to questions can be particularly telling. I sounded as evasive as my eight-year-old self when my sisters finally came home from school and asked me, "Why are you outside?" and I would reply, "Oh, I wanted to play in the yard." Now I was telling myself, *It's a freaking pandemic out there! It's natural to still be worried about my company.*

This inner evasiveness can be a clue to an idol lurking underneath. Idols resist being investigated. Like the craftsmen of Isaiah 41:5–7, idolatry deflects questions with, "It is good." We should be alerted when this happens, like when someone is too insistent in claiming, "It's all good. Nothing to see here." In my case, my next line of defense was to point out to God, *Look, I already realized I was looking to the company to bolster my Ideal Self as a successful entrepreneur. I already dealt with that. . . . It's all good . . . so . . . back off already!* But the Spirit kept probing for more layers. God wasn't done and wasn't satisfied with my deflections. I could not shake a sense of "holy unease." *Why? Why my company?*

During a prayer time, I finally submitted and asked God to show me what was going on. An image came to mind of a fortified castle brimming with defensive armament. Flying over the castle was a flag featuring one word—*provision.*

This was how I was led to the idol at the center of my rumination in the pandemic. For some time even before the crisis of the pandemic, God had been gently asking me to embrace a particular aspect of his love: God as my loving provider. My fears about not being provided for went deep and far back in my life. What was driving my anxious thoughts as a middle-aged man was actually not different from what drove my anxious thoughts as an eight-year-old. Underneath *Who gonna pay?* was the deeper question of *Who gonna care for me?* As a kid, I fretted, *If my parents don't ever come home, no one will be left to take care of me.* As a middle-aged man, I worried, *If my company doesn't survive, nothing will be left to take care of me.*

I was replaying my version of Isaiah 40–41. God was promising to love and care for me *through* any financial uncertainty. I wanted avoidance. I wanted *around* or *away.* I wanted certainty.

Deeply intertwined in the building of my company was the hidden drive to build an idol—something that could not be toppled, something that would avoid any possibility of loss. My company had become my idol, my ultimate provider. My rumination orbited around the pull of this nuclear idolatry.

Our strongest idols will promise avoidance of our most feared losses. My most feared loss will not necessarily be yours. I most fear the loss of provision; my wife most fears the loss of meeting the ideal; one of my best friends most fears the loss of belonging; another friend most fears the loss of independence. Idols come in so many forms because the anxieties they prey on come in so many forms. Each of us must engage in our own investigation with the help of the Spirit. This is why the author of Psalm 139 wisely asked God to search his anxious thoughts for "any idolatrous way in *me*" (CEB, emphasis added).

But—good news!—Psalm 139 also reminds us of the payoff. Locating that offensive way leads to "the way everlasting." Anxiety exposes our vulnerability to idolatry; it also presents the opportunity for repentance.

An activated desire for repentance is another indication we have accurately located a core idol. For me, this desire was expressed in grieving—the "godly sorrow" that "brings repentance that leads to salvation" (2 Corinthians 7:10). I'm not a teary person, but when I finally acknowledged to God that I had perverted his provision of my consulting practice into an idol that was replacing him, I wept. For days after my confession, the moment I turned to God in prayer, I bawled. The experience was both startling and wonderfully cathartic.

Stronger emotions swept through me as I committed myself to repentance. In prayer, I imagined that castle again and visualized myself lowering the drawbridge and the defiant flag. When I did, sorrow gave way to joy. The Spirit seemed to co-fashion my emotional experience from movie clips I had seen of the joyous celebrations of Allied soldiers finally liberating long-occupied European cities. That's what it felt like inside me.

It wasn't just emotional energy that got unlocked in the repentance. A level of unprecedented spiritual energy surged through my prayer life. For about two months after my repentance, the presence of God felt more tangible and accessible than ever before. I pray most often in my backyard, and in those months, it felt like what the ancient Celtic mystics call "a thin place," where the usual barriers to God are lowered. My backyard was pulsating with the energy of the Spirit.

This extraordinary spiritual season finally faded after a couple of months (why and when such seasons come and go is another of those mysteries of God's personal gift-giving nature). But through the following year and beyond, creative energy continued to explode out from me. Far more than simply surviving the pandemic, my consulting practice thrived and deepened in new ways. For instance, I developed a successful new program to train and mentor emerging nonprofit leaders of color. One of the most popular sessions is called "Managing Anxiety."

That session turned into an online video course on anxiety for Christian audiences that made the underlying biblical principles more explicit. And that course led to this book.

Creating videos on anxiety prepared me to respond when I sensed the Spirit calling me to help Christians handle their anxieties about the COVID-19 vaccine. I developed a set of videos to address their fears and eventually became a national spokesperson on the issue, appearing in national media and testifying before the US Senate.

A few years ago, I would have been wary about doing something this high-profile as a Christian in the public eye. I would have been less decisive, less willing to entertain such risky endeavors. Why? Because I would have been going around and around in my head with thoughts about how doing so might jeopardize my company's prospects in the Bay Area nonprofit market, which is highly secular and can have negative associations with anything to do with evangelical Christians. If I became nationally known as a spokesperson to evangelical Christians, well, *Who gonna pay?*

I would have worried about defending my little idol.

We all become our most powerful and creative selves when we become "undefended." We all have vast reserves of energy within us. Avoidance habits trap energy. Avoidance habits revolving around a nuclear core of idolatry especially trap a tremendous amount of emotional, spiritual, and creative energy. When we smash our idols, we are smashing the atomic core of our anxiety. The result can be an incredible release of productive energy.

What could that mean for you? Imagine all the energy now expended on defending against your feared losses. Imagine if that avoidance energy could instead be used by God for his purposes in the world.

CHAPTER 11

Getting Back What We Lose

A s you begin reading this chapter, I invite you to do a simple one-minute writing exercise. If you are a reader like me, you tend to skip over these kinds of exercises in books, so if you're tempted to do so here, I get it. However, please do consider doing this particular one now. Its applicability to anxiety may not be immediately apparent, but I promise that it is highly relevant. Taking sixty seconds to do this simple exercise now will significantly help you process the rest of this chapter.

Here's the exercise:

1. Take out a blank piece of paper and a pen.
2. Set your stopwatch app on your phone for sixty seconds.
3. For the next minute, free-associate and write whatever comes to your mind when you see the phrase "my eternal life."
4. Don't overthink it or worry about getting the "right" answer. This is a free-association exercise. Write down

whatever pops into your head, whether it is words, images, feelings, or whatever.

Have you done this? Okay, set aside this piece of paper for now. We'll return to it shortly.

The exercise should have already alerted you that in this chapter, we'll be making an unexpected connection—our thoughts about eternity and how they may influence our anxiety. For most, this connection will be brand-new because most Christians don't receive adequate teaching about eternity in the first place, much less learning about how this heady topic may be relevant to their current worries. If this connection is new for you, you may have to think more deeply about eternity and the actual promise of the resurrection than is customary. But it will be worth it because you are about to realize one of the most exciting and hopeful parts about being a Christian.

And to help you get started, here's a little story . . .

The Challenge

My younger daughter's eighteenth birthday party had come to an end. The guests said their goodbyes, and we began to clean up the kitchen and store the leftover sausages, chips, and drinks. My daughter looked at me and gestured toward the large metal bucket of melting ice that had held the drinks. I nodded, and we both rolled up our sleeves. No words needed. We had been doing this for years.

The Challenge was on.

The Challenge is simple. My daughter and I each put our arms into a bucket of ice-cold water. We stare at each other, and the person who can hold their arm underwater longest wins. I have no idea why I started the Challenge, but it is a tradition now.

I used to win easily every time. My daughter couldn't get much past the one-minute mark, which is when the arm starts to lose feeling—and it's not a comfortably numb feeling; it's an intense, burning sensation, like your arm is about to fall off. If you're new to ice baths, the feeling comes as a shock. You have a strong urge to yank your arm out of the water.

During these initial minutes, you're not in actual danger of permanent loss of limb or any lingering damage. That feeling of disembodiment is an interim state. It signals that you're on the verge of entering the restoration state. Professional trainers have athletes immerse limbs and even full bodies in ice baths for fifteen minutes. To gain the health benefits, you must hold on *through* that period when it feels like your body parts are dying.

"The first time you get in, it takes your breath away. It's quite an experience, but after 5 to 10 minutes it gets easier, especially if you breathe and relax," explains an expert from the National Strength and Conditioning Association. "The first few times it's super uncomfortable and painful, but you do build up a tolerance."[1]

The secret to nurturing this capacity to hold on is simultaneously simple and challenging: you must believe *you get back what you lose*. To hold on, you have to believe you'll get the feeling in your arm back and that the painful sensation of loss won't be permanent. This belief is an absolute prerequisite. Once you can grasp the truth that restoration will come on the other side of loss, you can anticipate its arrival amid the pain, and this anticipation builds your tolerance even more.

I hate to lose at any contest, so I kept this secret hidden from my daughter (look, we middle-aged men have to pick up "W's" where we can). Between one and two minutes, fear usually lodged in her worried eyes: *Maybe this is too much. Maybe I am going to lose my arm.* That's when I had her.

To her credit, she never backed down from the Challenge.

She was starting to creep up on the secret. Each time we played, she'd hold out a bit longer.

Which brings me back to her eighteenth birthday party. She seemed like she was particularly eager to throw down this time. We rolled up our sleeves and faced off across the icy waters. One minute passed. Two. Three. In her face, not a trace of doubt or uncertainty flashed. Four minutes passed. She held her arm steady. Positively nonchalant. Her newfound peacefulness threw me off my game, and I suddenly lost my mental hold on the secret. The burning sensation crawled from my arm into my shoulder, and the pain was all-consuming, pushing out my capacity to imagine what lay beyond it. I was starting to tell myself things like, *This game is stupid* and *I've got a lot of work to do.* I pulled out short of the five-minute mark. With a pumped (and numb) fist, my daughter celebrated her first victory over me in the Challenge.

When it comes to anxiety, we face a challenge far more momentous in consequences but similar in nature. We are called to hold on *through* the experience of loss. The secret to conquering this far weightier challenge is no different—we have to believe *we get back what we lose.* To hold on through loss, we must be able to anticipate the future restoration on the other side of loss. This is why holding a correct vision of eternity matters for anxiety. Eternity is when we get back what we lose. For Christians, the ultimate answer to life's anxiety is holding on to the promise of that future restoration. Therefore, gaining an accurate understanding of eternity—and the resurrection promise that opens the doorway to that future—matters deeply.

Holding On through Major Loss

This connection between anxiety and eternity is not commonly taught in Christian circles, but it is the key to unlocking fully the Anxiety Opportunity. So bear with me as we make this connection. Let's start by quickly reviewing how we got here. Recall that anxiety challenges us with our fear of some future loss. We are vulnerable to this fear because we live in the Now and Not Yet, where loss is unavoidable. We can try to delude ourselves that we can go *away* from or *around* loss, but elemental realities will frustrate any avoidance habit. Avoidance habits eventually backfire and increase anxiety.

This is the key insight of the Anxiety Formula (Anxiety = Loss × Avoidance). It is a mathematical way to represent this truth. Decreasing our avoidance will save us from unnecessarily multiplying the impact of Loss. For many everyday feared losses, lessening our avoidance may be enough to bring our anxiety to manageable levels. When our avoidance habits are defending idols, lessening those defenses can even unlock a significant amount of spiritual energy.

But what about truly major loss?

I'm talking about traumatic events like the loss of career, life savings, spouse, child, or, ultimately, one's own life. What addresses the moment when the doctor shares the results of a biopsy with a sober face and the words, "I'm afraid I have some bad news . . ."?

When facing major loss, we will be vulnerable to intense anxiety. The Anxiety Formula is a mathematical way to represent this truth as well. Even if we lower the avoidance quotient, the loss quotient remains. When the quantity of loss is objectively enormous by itself—like when we get that biopsy result—our overall anxiety will still be large.

We all live in the shadow of major loss. Death, the Loss of all losses, awaits us all. All of our lesser losses are encompassed in that final inevitable loss. The Anxiety Formula only encourages us to stare at this final outcome unblinkingly and not fall into futile and counterproductive habits of going away from or around loss. By itself, the Anxiety Formula can only encourage us to stop avoiding loss. By itself, the Anxiety Formula does not promise any restoration of our losses.

The Three Classic Formulas for Facing Loss

In this limitation, the Anxiety Formula is similar to the formulas that circulated in Jesus' lifetime. In his era, the Greco-Roman philosophers of the day offered three main options to face major loss: Stoicism, Epicureanism, and Platonism. These three formulas still dominate today, albeit in varying forms and names. In his day (and for today as well), Jesus opened up a brand-new doorway, a breathtaking alternative to these three options. To fully grasp how different this "Jesus opportunity" is, let's quickly review the three standard options.

Stoicism essentially urges followers to "do good despite loss." Stoicism affirms our calculations that death will inflict the loss of all, and it is useless to pretend otherwise. The follower of Stoicism finds meaning despite this inevitability by living a moral life in their allotted days. While ancient Stoicism rigorously defined "doing good" with a particular set of classic virtues, moderns tend to leave the definition to the individual. What is especially popular today are general virtues of other-centeredness—being loving, servant-hearted, kind, and the like. The modern Stoic message can be boiled down to this: "You are going to be eventually pushing up daisies, so while you still have breath, give flowers to others."

In comparison, *Epicureanism* encourages people to "enjoy life despite loss." The Epicurean also accepts the inevitability of loss but differs from the Stoic by emphasizing the goal of maximizing the enjoyment of their allotted days. In our era, the definition of enjoyment is again left to the individual and usually revolves around pleasurable sensory experiences. "Yes, you are going to be eventually pushing up daisies," says the modern Epicurean, "so make sure you smell the roses while you can."

Neither Stoicism nor Epicureanism offers any vision of a future beyond death, so both concentrate on maximizing something in our current lives, whether moral good or personal enjoyment. *Platonism* has a hazy notion of an afterlife, and here it bears a distant resemblance to Christianity. Indeed, that distant resemblance has led many Christians today to mistakenly conflate it with Jesus' vision of the future, leading to much confusion (more on that below).

Platonism is quite different from true Christianity. It claims, "Your loss is not real." Platonism describes our current life as only a shadowy reflection of what is ultimately real, which is a separate and higher spiritual plane. Our afterlife will be as disembodied souls that have escaped physical existence and will dwell in a higher spiritual plane. Platonism emphasizes that we should emotionally detach from our current loves, passions, desires, and sorrows as temporary and insubstantial. Our souls will leave all those bodily experiences behind. In this emphasis on soulful detachment from the things of this life and world, Platonism is most truly expressed today not in biblical Christianity but in Buddhism and other New Age philosophies. The simplistic summary of the Platonic way would be this: "Your physical body is going to be left behind pushing up daisies, so float above it all."

Despite the differences between Stoicism, Epicureanism, and Platonism, they all share a common answer to this question: *Do we get back what we lose?* For all three, the answer is a resounding no. These three options encourage us to go through loss by nurturing different holding capacities—holding on to our morality, to our enjoyment, or to our "souls." But none of these formulas promise to give back.

These three options do not give back what we most fear losing because they do not give back our bodies. All three options leave our bodies decomposing in the earth and pushing up daisies. True restoration of loss is impossible in these three options. Our bodies are inseparable from what we desire and love in life.

Think of your fear of major loss in your finances, relationships, or health. Don't all of those feared losses involve losing something intrinsic to your bodily existence? Your capacity to eat well and sleep comfortably that is threatened by financial loss; your bodily pleasure of sex and companionship that is lost when you encounter romantic loss; your interesting thoughts that disappear when your brain ceases receiving oxygen. Lose the body, and you lose what you desire. Lose the body, and you lose what you love.

The Jesus Formula

Against the backdrop of these primary options that dominated the ancient world and still do today, Jesus provides a radically different answer to the question, *Do we get back what we lose?* The actions, teaching, life, death, and resurrection of Jesus proclaim, "Yes! Yes! We get back what we lose—and more!" The resurrection promise of Jesus gives back because resurrection gives back our bodies. That is the definition of the word. Our bodies will not be pushing up daisies, but rather will be restored to us so we can once again smell the flowers, give them away to others, and run through (not float above) the fields. We get back what we lose—and more.

The "and more" comes in because Christian resurrection gives back *eternal* bodies. Our bodies will be raised in imperishable form (1 Corinthians 15:42–57). We are saved from all future loss as well. We get back what we lose and will get to keep it all because death itself will finally be defeated forever.

Furthermore, we get back even more from these eternal bodies. Jesus promises our resurrected, incorruptible bodies will be glorified (1 Corinthians 15:43; Philippians 3:21). The glorified body will achieve all that God ultimately intends for human capacity—a capacity sorely curtailed by the fall and its hand-maiden, death (Genesis 3:17–19).

The fall and the powers of death also obscure our perception of the glory present in fellow humans. The transfiguration—when the disciples received a sneak preview of Jesus' victory over death and his resulting glorified body—suggests we will feel awe when we finally encounter the glorified bodies of others (e.g., Matthew 17:1–9). With our new glorified bodies, people will be able to do more, and we will be able to recognize each other's glory with ever greater appreciation. The resurrection is the doorway to our Best Self.

We occasionally get a sneak preview of eternal glory. We have antecedents to what future glorification will be like. For instance, have you ever felt awe as you witnessed a magnificent athlete or transcendent musician perform their most amazing achievements? That is akin to what you will experience after the resurrection when you reencounter that nice but otherwise seemingly unremarkable elderly woman who has been greeting you with a smile every Sunday.[2] You will see the full glory of her hidden faithfulness to God, her silent devotion to God's people, and yes, her personal affection for you. And you will gasp in wonder. You will want to stand and applaud.

This resurrection promise of receiving eternal and glorified bodies sets Christianity utterly apart from Stoicism, Epicureanism, and Platonism. It is also what distinguishes a truly Christian approach to major loss and the accompanying anxieties. For instance, the Stoics, Epicureans, and Platonists would applaud how the previous chapters of this book exposed the futility of avoidance habits. "We're on the same page," I can hear them saying. "We also believe in looking at death squarely in the eyes." But they would recoil at the belief that we get back what we lose. They would describe this claim as foolish.

Similarly, today's secular mental health professionals would recognize many of the specific practices outlined thus far in this book. They would say, "Yes, we believe in the efficacy of interventions like mindful breathing, self-awareness, self-acceptance, and cognitive work." But "nurture a belief in the resurrection"? Secular mental health—even in its most "respectful of religion" form—can only nod politely but ultimately demur, "Uh, we don't do that sort of thing."

The resurrection of Jesus is "the thing" that defines Christians. As the apostle Paul says, if the resurrection is not true and "if only for this life we have hope in Christ, we are of all people most to be pitied" (1 Corinthians 15:19). On the resurrection we stake everything, including our ultimate approach to anxiety.

Christians hold on to more than morality, enjoyment, or our souls—we hold on to Someone. We hold on to Jesus, the one who conquered our ultimate opponent in the anxiety challenge: death itself, the Loss of all losses. Because Jesus was the only one to conquer that ultimate challenge, Jesus provides in his own resurrected body a unique answer to the question, *Do we get back what we lose?* To repeat, his answer is this: "Yes! We get back what we lose—and more! We also get eternal and glorified bodies."

But we have to learn to hold on while waiting. We get our eternal and glorified bodies when Jesus returns to restore all things. We are like children at home who cannot call a number to calculate the "day or hour" (Matthew 24:36) of this restoration and reunion. We are called to hold on to the promise that Jesus will pull into our driveways on that day, ready to give us our fully transformed and best selves.

Holding on for this promised event—especially through life's major losses—requires that we develop our holding capacity. Just as my daughter had to do in the Challenge, we have to learn to hold on to the promised restoration as we go through the experience of major loss. We cannot go *away* or *around*; we must hold on *through*. This holding capacity isn't easily acquired. We need Jesus to nurture this capacity in us, just as he did with his disciples.

The Grain of Truth

As Jesus neared his own encounter with death, he intensified his attempts to teach his disciples about his resurrection promise. One such attempt is found in John 12:23–28 (NTE). The passage is worth reading carefully, and we will unpack its meaning step-by-step.

> "The time has come," said Jesus in reply. "This is the moment for the son of man to be glorified. I'm telling you the solemn truth: unless a grain of wheat falls into the earth and dies, it remains all by itself. If it dies, though, it will produce lots of fruit. If you love your life, you'll lose it. If you hate your life in this world, you'll keep it for the life of the coming age.
>
> "If anyone serves me, they must follow me. Where I am, my servant will be too. If anyone serves me, the father will honour them.
>
> "Now my heart is troubled," Jesus went on. "What am I going to say? 'Father, save me from this moment?' No! It was because of this that I came to this moment. Father, glorify your name!"
>
> "I have glorified it," came a voice from heaven, "and I will glorify it again."

The scene opens with Jesus teaching a "solemn truth" about grain. As Jesus did so often in his brilliant teaching, he is here drawing on images that would be familiar to his audience in order to construct a metaphor that would open them to surprising new insights. In their context of subsistence farming, his listeners would all know that their future depended on the act of planting seed.

Jesus cleverly likens the burial of human beings to the planting of seed. Humans and seeds alike face the universal fate—falling into the earth and dying. The grain that "remains all by itself" can be interpreted in two compatible ways. This particular grain can be equated with an individual who does not believe there is anything more than this life (like the Stoic or the Epicurean). Such a life does not lead to anything beyond its short existence; it "remains all by itself." This solitary grain could also be likened to an individual who deludes herself that she alone ("all by itself") can avoid the universal destiny of every grain/human, which is burial/death. In this latter sense, we respond with the key insight from the Anxiety Formula: avoiding loss is futile. Avoidance literally (for a grain) and metaphorically (for a human) results in a fruitless outcome.

Jesus underlines the fruitlessness of striving to avoid loss by saying, "If you love your life, you'll lose it." "Love your life" doesn't refer to the way God wants us to properly value life and its many treasures—the people we love, thoughts we have, and experiences we feel. Read the Gospels, and you see in Jesus a human being fully alive and loving life in all its manifold and embodied glories. "Love your life" in this passage means idolatry—the way I was so committed to avoiding the loss of provision that I threw my anxious arms around my company instead of God. If you try to preserve your life by relying on idolatrous "love," Jesus is warning, you will lose everything. Avoidance via idols won't work, and you'll waste a great deal of your life. You will "lose your life" trying.

Like a good poet, Jesus employs dramatic contrast to depict an alternative to the false and fruitless "love" of our idols. He promises in John 12:25, "If you hate your life in this world, you'll keep it for the life of the coming age" (NTE). Jesus often uses the word *hate* as poetic hyperbole for repentance from "false loves," where we have elevated otherwise good things to idols. For example, when he says his followers must "hate father and mother" (Luke 14:26), he's talking about rejecting the way that fear of losing parental approval (which was especially powerful in ancient Jewish culture) can supplant allegiance to God. He wants our love of parents and everything else in our present life to be properly ordered loves and not be elevated into idols. To "hate your life in this world" means you can tolerate the loss of your idols.

Unfortunately, this verse about "hate your life in this world" in order to "keep it for the life of the coming age" has been misread to support a persistent misunderstanding in Christian circles today—namely, that our eternal state will be disembodied souls existing in some otherworldly plane called heaven. "Hate your life in this world" can be misunderstood as a Christianized version of the Platonic call to detach from earthly concerns and attach solely to one's eternal soul.

My conservative evangelical church imbued this message in me as a kid. I repeatedly heard some variation of "don't care too much about anything in this world because it's all going to burn." What would endure? Answer: our souls and heaven. And what would our souls be doing in heaven for all eternity? What kind of activity can disembodied "souls" do anyways? Here the answers provided to me as a kid got even fuzzier and less appealing, ranging from "floating about" (boring) to "resting" (really boring) to "eternally worshiping God" (which secretly sounded the most boring). For the latter, I could only imagine my dull Sunday church services, where I spent much of the time watching the clock wishing it would be over so I could make it home in time for the kickoff of a Chicago Bears football game. The vision of being stuck eternally in that state (without even a game to look forward to) was unappealing to say the least.

In my head, this spiritual vision was reinforced by other jumbled images of the afterlife that arose out of my consumption of popular culture. For example, the popular movie *Heaven Can Wait* came out when I was ten years old. The movie features the common recurring tropes in subsequent similar movies over the decades (such as Pixar's 2020 movie *Soul*). The lead character in *Heaven Can Wait* (played by Warren Beatty) dies and is transported to a separate realm called "heaven" (usually in an up-and-away physical trajectory), which is ethereal (marked by clouds or stars and other similar skyward characteristics).

The plot in all these movies rests on the Platonic sharp separation of one's ultimate self—the "soul"—from one's physical body. This separation is the basis for the "comedy of errors" element in these movies that invariably involves one's soul being swapped in and out of the shell of different bodies. Typically, the concluding plot resolution involves the character accepting one's final and eternal existence in "heaven" as a disembodied "soul."

This Platonic vision is deeply embedded in the popular imagination, and even young children are indoctrinated in it. I spent countless Saturdays watching Bugs Bunny cartoons where a character like Wile E. Coyote gets blown up spectacularly by TNT or has an Acme-branded anvil dropped on his head. Out of the debris, he sprouts wings, plays a harp, and floats into a "heaven" with its "pearly gates." Even as an adult, I find it difficult to get out of my head what I watched on TV as a kid.

How do you imagine your life in the coming age? Take out the piece of paper from the opening exercise and reread it. Here are three evaluative questions to pose to your vision:

1. **Who are you?** Are you a physical body with limbs and breath and beating heart? Or do you picture yourself as more akin to a disembodied "soul" floating about ethereally like a ghostly figure? Or is there even a clear answer to the Who question?

2. **Where are you?** Are you on earth with mountains, trees, flowers, oceans, and other aspects of creation? Are there objects like buildings, sculptures, and boats around you, along with other humanly constructed things? Or do you see insubstantial things, such as clouds and light? Are you in the air? Or is there even a recognizable answer to the Where question?

3. **What are you doing?** Are you eating, drinking, dancing, working, creating, and otherwise engaged in the activities you instinctively love to do? Are you doing them with the people you love? Or are you doing some activity that has little to no relevance to your lived experience? Or are you doing nothing? Is there even a coherent answer to the What question?

What was stored in your head? Perhaps you didn't even have a robust answer to the basic questions of Who, Where, and What. If so, this may indicate your imagination has been more shaped by the Stoic or Epicurean vision, which leaves the vision of eternity entirely blank. Stoicism and Epicureanism have affected many contemporary expressions of Christianity, where teaching focuses much more on moral behavior (Stoicism) or personal fulfillment (Epicureanism) than on the resurrection.

It is striking how often Easter sermons reduce the resurrection to a metaphor for moral reform or renewed fulfillment in this life and bypass the actual meaning of the resurrection and its promise of eternal and glorified bodies. When it comes to imagining your eternal state, Christianity as "do the right thing" or "get the life you've always wanted" results in blank pages or at least extreme fuzziness.

Or does your imagined eternal state more resemble the Platonic vision of being disembodied and detached from our world? If you detect the influence of Platonic imagery, you would not be alone. If I had done this chapter's opening writing exercise as a college student, the Platonic version of eternity would have been in my paper. Fortunately, as a graduate student, I had the privilege of learning directly from the biblical scholar N. T. Wright. His lectures—and his many books that I've since read—transformed my vision of eternity. His book *Surprised by Hope: Rethinking Heaven, the Resurrection, and the Mission of the Church* is a particularly masterful and accessible correction of the Christian imagination pertaining to what happens after death.[3]

Wright documents in this book and in other writings Platonism's role in the history of the church and how it distorted the Christian teaching about eternity. There are complex reasons for this distortion, but the brief historical explanation is this: as Christianity spread into the Greco-Roman world in the first millennium, leading thinkers such as Augustine sought to make the gospel relevant to existing pagan worldviews, especially Platonism. As I've written in a previous book, Augustine for the most part achieved this brilliantly, specifically showing how the deep desires of Platonism can only be satisfied by Christ.[4]

But Augustine's efforts (and the efforts of his intellectual successors) were not immune from the ever-present danger facing evangelists—distorting the gospel for the sake of cultural relevance. Seeking to be relevant to the Platonic worldview, the Christian vision of the future Not Yet (especially in the early medieval era and at the popular level) itself began to be tinged with a greater emphasis on disembodied souls and a heaven disconnected from earthly realities.

The Platonic vision gained a particular foothold in Christianity because it does contain a grain of truth. The "go away to heaven" and "disembodied soul" version of the future could possibly describe the interim state between death and resurrection. For those who die before Jesus' return—which will accomplish the resurrection of the dead—there is a period of waiting for our new bodies. The precise nature of our self in that interim state is clouded in mystery (Are we conscious? Do we act and move about?), but it seems we are at peace in God's presence. In that temporary sense, we do "go away to heaven" and perhaps exist as "disembodied souls." We don't know what that interim state will feel like because the Bible doesn't provide specifics.[5]

Regardless of speculations about the interim state, it is an *interim* state. Even if our temporary state is disembodied, that is the state of *waiting*. It is not the eternal future we are waiting and holding on for in the ultimate sense. Just like I got thrown off my game in the ice bucket challenge by focusing on the initial feeling of disembodiment, we will get thrown off if we overly focus on that interim state.

The confusion between the interim state and the final state is frequently found in funeral services. And with some deaths, the disembodied vision of the future can seem appealing in the moment. A few years ago, I witnessed my father suffer an arduous and painful death from chronic kidney disease. In such cases, disembodiment can indeed seem like an immediate relief.

At the memorial service, the pastor of my parents' church patted me on the arm.

"He's enjoying his eternal rest." His voice was soft as he situated himself next to me in the pew. "He's in his final home with God now."

His encouragement may have been well-intentioned, but it was not biblically accurate. My dad's state of "rest" was only his interim state; he still awaits his "final home." This is not just a theological nitpick; this is a matter of deep pastoral importance. As much as I was grateful that my dad was no longer suffering, my stronger desire was to have him back. I am still a son who has lost his father. What I lost was the man whose physical arrival in the driveway comforted me and who patted me on my back after disastrous Little League games. I most needed to hear that I will one day get that man back in all his embodied and newfound glory.

I smiled wordlessly at the well-meaning pastor. It was not the time to engage in a theological discussion, but I did my own internal correction. In that moment and in others like it, I've tried to excise those phrases from my mental vision of eternity. I have become more conscious of what I say when consoling others who have lost their loved ones. What we put on our mental pages matters. It mattered to how I held on through the loss of my dad. It will matter to how I hold on through the loss of my own life. It will matter for how you hold on through your major losses.

For many Christians, the vision of eternity is fuzzy because we've confused the interim state (which is indeed fuzzy in Scripture) with our permanent future. We are meant to focus much more on our permanent future. I believe this is why Scripture provides relatively few clues about the interim state and leaves it a bit vague compared to much more vivid depictions of the final destination. It seems that the biblical authors did not want to distract us and throw us off our game. Biblical descriptions of the final state (such as the beautifully vivid, long passage found in Isaiah 60–66) portray our ultimate destiny in thoroughly embodied terms. We are meant to look past the interim state and anticipate the restoration beyond.

All of this matters for anxiety. To hold on *through* our feared losses, we have to hold on to some vision of the future. What you wrote in the free association exercise represents what you will be reaching for in your mind when your doctor shares the bad news. If your page was blank, fuzzy, or incorrect, you will be unprepared. We all must allow Jesus to fill our imagination with his truth. A correct imagination matters.

Each anxiety we face is an opportunity for Jesus to correct our picture of eternity and reinforce our hold on his truth. The next chapter will explore further how we cooperate with Jesus in this process.

CHAPTER 12

Throughlines to Eternity

If the previous chapter's discussion of eternity and resurrection felt new and perhaps disorienting, you shouldn't feel bad. You are not alone. The Gospels describe the disciples as confused initially by the new promise introduced by Jesus' resurrection. They needed time to work it all out, especially with the further help of Jesus. You also are not to blame. Those of us responsible for Christian education (like I was for many years) haven't done enough to help you grasp the full truth of resurrection, much less connect it to anxiety.

But whatever you are feeling, please don't give in to the temptation that these topics are just reserved for the theological "experts" to grasp and not relevant to you. Jesus wants you to realize that through his resurrection, he has opened up for you a doorway to eternity. Accurately envisioning this doorway will change everything in your life, including your anxiety. In fact, your anxiety can serve as a key to unlock this new vision.

Jesus Reunites with His Anxious Disciples

Jesus sought to correct his disciples' vision, and he began with their anxiety. In Luke 24, the resurrected Jesus approaches them as they huddle together in Jerusalem. They are afraid because the crucifixion has dealt an enormous loss to the disciples, and even more losses loom in the future. They staked their futures on their beloved Master, but Jesus had been killed and they fear they will be next. Naturally, the disciples are thrown into a state of intense anxiety, as all the Gospels describe.

Zero in on the story in Luke 24:36–43 as the resurrected Jesus reappears to the disciples. What is striking is that this reunion initially fails to reassure them, but rather momentarily worsens their condition. The text reports that they were "startled and frightened and thought they saw a spirit" (v. 37 ESV). The disciples are, of course, startled because they hadn't expected Jesus to appear. But why are they frightened by their vision of Jesus? Why do they not receive reassurance from this vision of Jesus, as Jesus must have intended them to? Answer: because *they thought they saw a spirit.* They mistakenly thought this presence was a disembodied spirit (other translations use the term *ghost*). Like many Christians today, they did not grasp the bodily nature of the resurrection.

In other words, the disciples initially didn't think they were getting back what they lost. All of their treasured experiences with Jesus were thoroughly embodied. He was someone who walked, drank, ate, and sailed with them physically. The Jesus they loved had a body, but this ghostly being (in their mistaken view) does not. Therefore, they fail to meaningfully connect the dots. The disciples in this moment are like many Christians today. Their conception of what comes after death is something fuzzy, foreign, and disconnected from their most treasured experiences. Hence, their anxiety is unassuaged.

We are no different from the disciples. Imagine how my eight-year-old latchkey self would have felt if my parents' vehicle pulled into the driveway, the car door opened, and two ethereal spirits floated out to greet me. Wouldn't that kind of reunion frighten me, just like it did the disciples?

Pay attention to what Jesus does next:

> And he said to them, "Why are you troubled, and why do doubts arise in your hearts? See my hands and my feet, that it is I myself. Touch me, and see. For a spirit does not have flesh and bones as you see that I have." And when he had said this, he showed them his hands and his feet. (Luke 24:38–40 ESV)

Jesus addresses their fears by emphasizing the bodily nature of the resurrection. Jesus connects the dots for them. He asks them to touch his new hands and feet, just as they did in the past. The reunion that reassures us—at any age and in any era—is a *bodily reunion*.

Emphasizing the bodily nature of resurrection is of the utmost importance in Jesus' response to why they are "troubled" and why "doubts arise" in their hearts. He is not picking theological nits. He is getting at the heart of human anxiety. He is answering for his disciples the fundamental question, *Do we get back what we lose?*

"See my hands and my feet" is how the disciples are reassured that the one they lost is being fully given back to them—"that it is I myself." His hands and his feet bore the marks of major loss—the brutal crucifixion that took Jesus away from the disciples. Therefore, the fact that Jesus is back in flesh and bones that the disciples can touch and see confirms they are getting back what—or more precisely Whom—they had lost. He is drawing a new line for his disciples, a line that runs from their treasured past, goes *through* death and the loss of those treasures, and ends in the restoration of all that had been lost. Establishing this line is precisely how Jesus addressed his disciples' anxiety.

Jesus seeks to draw this same line for you. He wants to do this because a true answer to our anxiety must also be a picture of a future that has some recognizable antecedent in our current reality. We also need to connect the dots, with a line that runs from all that we fear losing, through death, and on to our future restoration. This is why the Platonized Christian vision of disembodied souls in heaven does not adequately assure us in our anxiety. It lacks any recognizable antecedent in our embodied experiences of what we desire and what we fear losing. To repeat, the "souls going away to heaven for eternity" vision does *not* give us back what we lose. Instead, it offers a substitute that is foreign, fuzzy, and ultimately false.

Why Throughlines Matter

What Jesus accomplished in Luke 24 reminds me of the concept of a "throughline"—a key idea that comes from the field of narrative drama. Accomplished storytellers recognize that the audience will only trust a story if they believe (even subconsciously) that the characters are staying true to their underlying nature. Konstantin Stanislavski, a famous proponent of method acting, described the concept of throughline by explaining that "actors should not only understand what their character was doing, or trying to do . . . in any given unit, but should also strive to understand the through line which linked these objectives together and thus pushed the character forward through the narrative."[1]

The throughline is usually an underlying motivation that

connects the character's past, present, and future. The moment the audience thinks, *So-and-so wouldn't have done that!* because this new action was so disconnected from what came before it, the story starts to ring false. By the way, this doesn't mean that stories can't contain surprises—quite the contrary, the best stories must include unexpected twists, but the twist must make sense by remaining connected to the throughline.

Many books or movies feature the special power of a throughline that is getting back a desired objective that was lost (or feared to be lost). In *The Da Vinci Code*, the throughline is Robert Langdon's desire to recover his innocent status. In *The Fast and Furious* movie franchise, the throughline is the heroes' desire for their nonbiological "family" to be reunited (which is why seemingly dead characters keep getting resurrected in the never-ending string of sequels). In *The Lord of the Rings*, a key throughline for the hobbits is their desire to return to the Shire.

Throughlines that authentically motivate the characters—and ring true to the audience—must pay off on this desire for restoration in some coherent fashion (which can still involve the element of surprise). If *The Lord of the Rings* ended with the hobbits never returning to the Shire but instead, say, opening a bed-and-breakfast in Mordor, the story would seem utterly incoherent.

This is why the view of heaven presented to me as a child was so unmotivating, boring, and ultimately incoherent. That envisioned conclusion had no throughline that gripped me. I had no antecedent desire anywhere close to floating to heaven on angelic wings (my childhood desire was to become a fighter pilot, so if the envisioned angel wings were going to be equipped with heat-seeking missiles, I might have been interested). I never played the harp, I never feared losing the ability to play the harp, and the prospect of now having to play the harp for eternity sounded like an endless version of those awful piano recitals I endured as a kid. Similarly, the prospect of being stuck in a worship service singing the same song over and over did not pay off on any strongly felt desire. Deep down, even if I couldn't admit it at the time, something about this story of eternity rang false. Or at least it rang weak. The motivational pull of eternity remained weak into my adulthood—until my mind began to be corrected by a more biblically accurate vision of eternity.

Our Throughline to Our Best Self

Jesus intends to give a motivating throughline to his anxious followers. Let's turn back to the story in Luke 24. As Jesus shows the disciples his hands and feet and asks them to touch him in his restored physical being, their emotional state begins to change dramatically. They start to shift from their initial troubled and doubting state. Luke describes the process—and how Jesus reinforces the change—in a beautiful fashion:

> And while they still disbelieved for joy and were marveling, he said to them, "Have you anything here to eat?" They gave him a piece of broiled fish, and he took it and ate before them. (Luke 24:41–43 ESV)

The disciples are starting to connect the dots. From their initial fear, they now "disbelieved for joy and were marveling." I love how Jesus keeps coloring the lines in a way both ordinary and touchingly intimate. He then asks the kind of ordinary question posed only by longtime roommates to one another or by children to their parents: "Have you anything here to eat?" He eats a leftover piece of fish, deliberately doing it "before them" to demonstrate the truth that resurrection means getting back a body that chews, tastes, and swallows.

Jesus shows his anxious disciples that he had gotten back his body because what they had lost were treasured experiences with Jesus that were thoroughly bodily in nature. They've suffered the traumatic loss of their beloved teacher with whom they walked, talked, and, yes, ate. Late-night meals shared together after a long day (it was "late in the evening" according to Luke 24:29) must have been precisely the kind of intimate gathering they had enjoyed with Jesus countless times.

The shared meal summed up what they had lost. So the post-resurrection Jesus deliberately hosts a little impromptu dinner as a throughline to eternity, showing them that the resurrection gives them back what they lost. Jesus will throw another similar dinner in John 21:1–14, when he hosts another postresurrection reunion (this time in a beachside location) with bread and fish that he himself cooks. Jesus consistently weaves his throughline to eternity with parties.

The disciples will need to hold on to this throughline. Jesus predicted their future in the "grain of wheat" exchange: "Whoever serves me must follow me; and where I am, my servant also will be. My Father will honor the one who serves me" (John 12:26). Almost all of his disciples would face painful persecution and death, like Jesus had. If they were to share in a similar loss of life, they would need to share in the promise of a similar restoration of life—that the Father will honor them. They will need to remember these intimate dinner reunions with Jesus.

To restate our chapter 1 analysis of the "clobber verse" of Philippians 4:6, the encouragement to "not be anxious about anything" only makes sense because a couple of verses earlier, Paul had presented a succinct statement of the Christian hope for eternity:

> But our citizenship is in heaven. And we eagerly await a Savior
> from there, the Lord Jesus Christ, who, by the power that

enables him to bring everything under his control, will transform our lowly bodies so that they will be like his glorious body. (Philippians 3:20–21)

The throughline to this ultimate outcome of our bodies becoming "like his glorious body" underwrites the Philippians 4:6 practical encouragement. The biblical reason to not be anxious is not "because you won't suffer loss," but rather "because you will be restored to glory." I cannot emphasize this enough to my fellow Christians: we are promised resurrection, not loss avoidance. Indeed, resurrection is the opposite of loss avoidance, because we only get to resurrection by going through loss first.

To hold on through our major losses, we must hold on to the resurrection throughline. Resurrection distinguishes a Christian approach to anxiety from all other alternatives. Resurrection is what makes the Christian approach to anxiety, in my view, the best one on offer. It is best because it is the doorway to our best self, our glorified self.

Our Throughline to Our Best World

In the end, our bodies will be restored in the same way Jesus' body was restored. We will participate in his glorious new capacity. We will be given our true best selves. In eternity, these glorious new capacities will be exercised in the way we care for a redeemed world. Note in Philippians 3:20–21 how the promised resurrection of the body is intertwined with the promised redemption of the world. The same resurrection power of Jesus will transform everything in the world "by the power that enables him to bring *everything* under his control" (v. 21, emphasis added). This future reality where all things on earth are restored is what Jesus calls "the kingdom of heaven." This kingdom compels our highest allegiance and constitutes what Paul calls our true "citizenship in heaven."

Here is another key correction for Platonized Christians. The movement of the kingdom of heaven is not that we escape this earth *away* to heaven but that Jesus will bring heaven *to* earth. Note the flow of the passage: "And we eagerly *await* a Savior *from* there [heaven], the Lord Jesus Christ" (Philippians 3:20, emphasis added). In the Now, this future restoration of the entire world is being held securely in heaven by Jesus. The Not Yet is when Jesus returns to earth to reunite heaven to this earth and thus transform "everything" on earth. Our best selves will be doing our best work in our best earth.

The intimate reunion of Jesus and his disciples celebrated by a meal of grilled fish prefigures a cosmic reunion between the kingdom of heaven and the earth celebrated at the wedding feast of the Lamb. This is why Jesus taught his disciples to pray to the Father that his kingdom would come on this earth (see Matthew 6:10), not "Father, get us out of here!" This is also why the final scenes of the entire Bible in Revelation 21–22 are depicting the kingdom of heaven descending to earth and transforming our broken earthly realities (see especially Revelation 21:1–4). Heaven comes to us on earth; we don't go away from the earth to heaven.

Jesus seeks to address our anxiety by filling our minds with both the promise of the resurrection of our bodies and the promise of the redemption of this earth. The latter must be included because we also fear major losses suffered by the wider world our bodies inhabit.

In 2021, a landmark global survey of youth ages sixteen to twenty-five revealed that 60 percent are feeling "very worried" or "extremely worried" about climate change, with 45 percent reporting that such worries "impacted their daily lives."[2] My daughter is one of these individuals, and this anxiety is real in her and her friends. Her generation suffers from a profound sense of hopelessness that can be paralyzing.

Even if climate change is not your most pressing worry, you are immersed constantly in media coverage about other anxieties in the economy, in the broader culture, in national politics, and in global issues. News today is all about stoking fears of loss in the wider world because media companies garner more clicks when they tap into our anxieties. Ask yourself this simple question: *After scrolling through my newsfeed, does my anxiety level tend to go up or down?* Multiple studies show that news consumption increases anxiety, especially during times of uncertainty such as the pandemic[3] and presidential elections.[4] This is when we fear major losses suffered by the world.

We desperately need to be reminded that Jesus will restore our world from its grievous losses. The notion that "none of this matters because it's all going to burn" is not only biblically incorrect, but it also rings emotionally hollow and callous for people (like my daughter) who care deeply about this world. Indeed, the religious belief that we are going to "go away to heaven" and leave behind this world is literally a theological *away* move—a way to distract people and to underwrite widespread avoidance of the real pain in the world.

People need real hope in order to sustain an ongoing engagement with the real suffering occurring in the world. This is especially true when we recognize that our own tiny efforts can hardly make a dent in avoiding major loss (such as with the issue of climate change). We must believe that the kingdom of heaven will eventually come. Our small efforts only serve as signposts pointing to that future, as creative and suggestive throughlines to eternity. Jesus—not our puny efforts—will raise the dead and restore all things. In the absence of this kingdom imagination that informs all social and political activity, Christian activists will be sorely tempted to view their own efforts and immediate outcomes as the "be all and end all." Within a constricted imagination, we will swing back and forth between despairing paralysis and cataclysmic extremism. We will either pull out of a current fight (because we believe it is hopeless) or inappropriately stake everything on the narrow outcome of a current fight (because we've lost sight of the broader and guaranteed future). Either way, anxiety will have defeated us.

If Christians are going to hold on through the major losses suffered by our bodies and our world, we need to live, act, and suffer while envisioning our eternal future. We need imaginations filled with compelling descriptions of the resurrection of our bodies and the redemption of the earth. To repeat, compelling descriptions of eternity must contain some throughline to our embodied existence in this concrete world. Eternity must be connected to some antecedent experience of what we desire and fear losing.

This is Jesus' point in his "grain of wheat" metaphor. The grain mysteriously contains within itself the harvest. Therefore, to anticipate the harvest, look at the grain. The grain holds the raw ingredients for imagining the harvest.

For the former athlete who is tragically wasting away from Lou Gehrig's disease, their vision of eternity is not found in "floating away to heaven," but rather in the memories of the glory they felt running free on the playing field. For the environmental activist, their vision of redemption is not sustained by "it's all going to burn," but instead is nurtured by the sights, sounds, and smells of their favorite hike through the forest.

How do we nurture our imaginations so that we more strongly grasp this throughline to eternity that Jesus has provided? What new practices are needed? This practical question is the subject of our next chapter.

CHAPTER 13

Nurturing Our Imagination

The most life-changing truths are the ones that reshape not just our thinking but also our imaginations. The last several chapters have sought to lay out the truth of the resurrection and how it radically reshapes our thinking about anxiety. Practically speaking, how do we allow this truth of Jesus to sink deeper and reach into our imagination? Let's explore this question with the guidance of the Master himself.

"Harvest Festivals" and the Get Back

Like any great teacher, Jesus nurtured the imagination of his disciples by starting with what was already in their minds. The first-century Jewish conception of individual eternal life (in the sense of "everlasting life after death") was somewhat fuzzy, but vivid visions of God's corporate restoration of his people Israel did exist. If Jesus had given his disciples a version of the writing exercise I gave you at the beginning of chapter 11 and asked them to write about what God's restoration of Israel would be like, many likely would have written down, "God's restoration will be kind of like . . . the harvest." In an ancient agricultural society like Israel, where survival depended on what happened after the labor of planting and the months of anxious waiting, the harvest symbolized what it meant to *get back*. This annual expectation naturally served as a potent image for when God would make everything right once and for all.

This imaginative association between the harvest and ultimate restoration by God was reinforced powerfully through the "harvest festivals." The Israelite culture (both in Jesus' day and still today) celebrated three such harvest festivals: *Sukkot* (or Festival of Tabernacles; Leviticus 23:33–34), *Shavuot* (or Festival of Weeks; Leviticus 23:15–16), and especially *Pesach* (or Passover; Leviticus 23:5). These three festivals were large-scale celebrations involving food, reunions, dancing, and travel. Historically, many Jews would together undertake a pilgrimage to Jerusalem to attend the Passover festival, making it a time of heartfelt reunion.

These highly sensory and physical experiences were meant to intensify people's anticipation of God's ultimate restoration. This is why Jesus' timing for his entry into Jerusalem right before the Passover festival was so explosive. It whipped up the masses to believe that Jesus was indeed the Messiah who would give back to Israel the political independence it had lost to Rome. Their instinctive reaction shows how the regular celebration of such harvest festivals had nurtured the Jewish imagination of their future restoration. Jesus must dramatically rework this existing imagination for his disciples to expand their vision beyond the narrow political lines of the day. But he draws on the harvest festival as raw material to form their vision of God's fuller restoration.

What is the equivalent of the harvest festival in our minds

today? What can the Spirit of Jesus draw on to form our resurrection hope? If Jesus were to craft the equivalent of the "grain of wheat" metaphor for us today, what would he use to spark our imagination of what it feels like to *get back*?

I'm talking about the equivalent of the harvest festival as *festival*—an embodied, multisensory celebration we share with others. In the long centuries of Christian tradition, an obvious candidate has been the wedding festival. Weddings are meant to not just celebrate something significant happening to two individuals now—although it is that. Weddings are also meant to give us embodied foretastes of the "marriage" between God and his people, the final union between the kingdom of heaven and earth. Our wedding feasts are meant as signposts to the final wedding feast of the Lamb (Revelation 19:7–10).

The intended throughlines are rich and evocative. Desires are heightened. The eagerness of the couple to finally have a new bodily experience together (that is, if and when sexual abstinence before marriage still retains both assumed status and spiritual meaning) is a throughline to our longing for our new glorified bodies. For the extended family, the wedding festival was the occasion of many long-awaited reunions pointing to the final reunion. For all the guests, the anticipation of the special feast was meant as a throughline to the anticipation of God's abundance in the final feast. In these and other ways, the wedding festival was meant to fill people's minds with a rich stock of images, so if they were ever asked to free-associate about eternal life, they could write, "It will be kind of like . . . a wedding."

Today, these imaginative throughlines have mostly been severed. One hangs by a thread in the traditional liturgy via the phrase (as found in the *Book of Common Prayer*) that marriage "signifies to us the mystery of the union between Christ and his Church."[1] But more and more weddings have eliminated even

169

that reference, and those that retain it usually pass by it quickly without much elaboration.

More tellingly, the "festive" part of most Christian weddings lacks any intentional throughline to eternity. In my pastoral career, I officiated a number of weddings. When it came to the actual banquet and party (truth be told, this was the more highly anticipated event for many guests such that I made sure my homily was very brief), it was difficult to locate even a slight evocation of the wedding feast of the Lamb. I felt this absence most keenly during the wedding banquet toasts, the time of the party when participants have the most explicit opportunity to define the meaning of the event. Wedding toasts are now almost entirely focused on the wonderful qualities of the couple. It is as if all the signposts are pointing to each other, with no reference to anything beyond, and certainly not to our shared final destination.

I know I run the risk of coming off as a theological fuddy-duddy, especially because we lack good models for how such events can still be fully festive and also recover their God-intended signposting function. Nobody, even a theological nerd like me, wants to turn a party into a long lecture. But if we are to restock our imaginations with eternity, we need to creatively experiment with refashioning our festivals as *signposts*.

Jody and I recently held such an experiment. We hosted a large party to celebrate our twenty-fifth anniversary and renew our marriage vows. More than one hundred of our closest friends and family joined us, some of them traveling great distances. Together we savored carefully prepared dishes and well-chosen wines. On the dance floor, the guests moved in unison to the "electric slide" and the beat of other 1980s dance music. At the end of the evening, Jody and I hugged our adult daughters, their heads resting on our shoulders. It was gloriously festive.

Yet for us, the most meaningful part of the party—the part

Jody and I spent the longest time planning—was the dinner toast part. We included the usual practice of guests toasting us and our qualities, and that was lovely. And then we invited our guests to look around the room at one another and reflect on their feelings for others, and we gave them time to mingle around the room and toast one another. In inviting them to this practice, I tried to direct our minds forward to eternity. I spoke briefly about the meaning of the "till death do us part" phrase in the wedding vows Jody and I had repeated earlier that night and about how all our relationships serve as a throughline to a greater and more lasting glory beyond death. It was our version of Jesus' dinner reunions (only with more varied catering options).

It was a risk to depart from usual toasting conventions and, even for an ex-pastor, to evoke death and eternity so deliberately in the middle of a party. But as our guests spread across the room, we heard the buzz of shared words and the tinkling of glasses and witnessed long and tight embraces. The room vibrated with love and joy. As many guests shared with us afterward, many of us felt like we were indeed glimpsing a preview of the wedding feast of the Lamb.

At this point, you may be wondering why a book about anxiety has suddenly become a book about party planning. The two are not as disconnected as you may think. Just as the disciples' loss could be summed up as losing the intimacy of the shared meal with Jesus, pretty much every one of my most feared losses can be summed up as losing something that was present at our party. I fear my heart might give out before I get to celebrate my fiftieth wedding anniversary with Jody. I worry where our daughters will be, whether they'll be okay, and whether they'll be at my side. I fret about whether my aging body will still be able to do things like the electric slide. I am anxious about several guests—including my mom—who already have received difficult news or diagnoses from their doctor. There will come a day when I will lose all these treasures.

When that day looms and my anxieties increase, I need to hang on through loss. To hang on through loss, I need to hang on to a throughline. The disciples hung on to the memory of their postresurrection dinner reunions (these events were retold enough to be recorded in multiple gospel texts).

To hang on through loss, we need to hang on to a throughline.

Similarly, my memories of the party will serve as a throughline to the Day beyond when we all get back what we lose—and more. This is why I periodically replay the images of this celebration. Photos of the event repeat on my screen saver. A framed poster bearing the handwritten wishes of attendees sits outside my bedroom to greet me every morning. I replay these images to stockpile material in my mind for the Spirit of Jesus to draw on to remind me what the final feast will be like. I look at those images and try to envision how that festival will be "more"—tastes of even more delicious food, expressions of love that have matured and deepened even more, and yes, even more dancing. By the way, in eternity, we will still be grooving to '80s dance music because as everyone knows, it is the best dance music *ever*.

What are your "harvest festivals?" What heightens your desire for ultimate restoration? Consider all the celebratory events of our lives—landmark birthdays, long-anticipated reunions, key anniversaries, and the like. I believe they all contain within them foretastes of eternity. They represent what we most long to *get back* in the end. They are our closest signposts and throughlines to glory. I don't have all the answers on how to refashion them so that they better serve their full God-intended functions (and this really isn't meant to be a book about event planning).

I do invite those who have the gift of hospitality to take

more risks and be more creative in subtly repositioning how our lowercase parties can point to *the* Party.[2] But for the rest of us who cannot redesign the festivals themselves, perhaps we can consciously reposition our remembrance of those festivals to be more than exercises in nostalgia. Nostalgia is pointing back to and longing for the past. I invite you to look at a treasured photo as also a signpost pointing forward, whetting your appetite for the time when you will get back the deepest treasure embedded in that photo. Ask the Spirit of Jesus to use that photo as a preview of the Not Yet.

As helpful as I hope private practices like viewing photos can be, I believe the onus for reform rests most urgently with Christian leaders who plan our most regular "harvest festival"— our Sunday church gatherings, especially in our songs and Communion experience. Here we desperately need the renewed imaginations of our pastors, worship leaders, musicians, liturgists, and songwriters.

I'm not talking about making our worship services slicker in production. While better production values might have helped a bit to alleviate the boredom of my childhood experiences on Sunday, that wasn't the real problem. What was missing was a compelling throughline to eternity. As an adult pastor, I remember preaching on the resurrection once and being sobered in realizing how difficult it was to construct a worship set with songs about the true Christian hope of resurrection (note: my church's worship drew from the CCLI stock of songs). Even for songs including a resurrection theme, it was often (like the Easter sermons I mentioned earlier) reduced to a metaphor for a current-day emotional experience, change in moral behavior, or purely interior spiritual experience. We desperately need more worship songs with lyrics celebrating the actual resurrection of bodies and the redemption of the concrete world. At any given

Sunday church service, people are facing concrete losses—imminent divorces, medical diagnoses, unemployment, and other losses. When worlds have been shaken and major losses loom, people are grasping for something to hold on to. We must give them the right lines.

"Grainy" Images of Loss

In their need to grasp the truth that *they would get back what they lost*, the disciples were already equipped by their harvest festivals to imagine the *we get back* part. What they were wholly unprepared for was connecting God's restoration to the *what we lose* part. The idea that the Messiah had to go through loss in order to achieve the restoration was so anathema to the disciples that it provoked the sharpest conflict between them and Jesus (see Matthew 16:21–24).

This is why Jesus' "grain of wheat" teaching reveals a brilliant teacher at work. He is taking the well-known imagery of the harvest and drawing a throughline to the more obscure imagery of the grain that "falls into the earth and dies" (John 12:24 ESV). The image of the *get back* is tied to the image of *what we lose*. In his metaphor, Jesus pulls this throughline so tautly that the connection is inescapable. The underlying logic is unassailable: just as you cannot get the harvest without the grain's burial, you cannot imagine resurrection unless you can properly imagine death.

Like the disciples, we also resist images of death, albeit for different reasons. The disciples did not want to connect death with their expectations for the Messiah. We today don't want to connect with death at all. Our modern world is filled with entire industries that promote the avoidance of death. Think of the billions of dollars spent every year on avoiding the inevitable loss of life through expensive (and often dehumanizing) medical procedures near the end of life. This medicalizing of death takes place away from our homes at the hospital, so most children never get exposed to the dying process. If our era has stripped our "harvest festivals" from their signposting function, we have largely banished our "grain events" from public view entirely.

Even the pathway to our inevitable death is kept out of sight. Consider the billions of dollars spent every year on cosmetic procedures attempting to camouflage our bodily decay. Or the billions of dollars the travel industry spends to promote to seniors the illusion that the tail end of life is an endless string of cruises. Our modern Western culture, more than any other culture in human history, goes to extreme lengths to avoid contemplating the Loss of all losses. This same modern Western culture is probably also the most psychologically anxious culture in human history. The Anxiety Formula tells us this is not a coincidence.[3]

In the "grain of wheat" metaphor, Jesus insists if we wish to hold on to the throughline to eternity, we have to follow that line through death. We have to imagine death enough to see it not as some utterly aversive event we go *away* from or *around*, but instead as something recognizable enough to go *through*. When we thoughtfully stock our minds with images of death, we give the Spirit of Jesus the raw material to draw mental throughlines from death to resurrection.

This intention goes all the way back to the early church. Several years ago, I toured the catacombs surrounding Rome. The catacombs are underground tombs that served as community cemeteries, and the early church famously gathered there for worship services and shared meals. My tour revealed something fascinating. Like many, I had thought the early Christians used the catacombs as underground hiding places to escape persecution. Historians and archaeologists now realize they were meeting there not to avoid the threat of death; instead, they were using the catacombs to be nearer to death.[4]

Christians wanted to stay close to the bodies of their recently deceased loved ones, so they dug out areas—little rooms—to be near them. And *close* is the key adjective, for these meeting rooms placed the visitors right next to the stored corpses (wrapped and prepared to prevent the stench of decomposition). Scholars now believe these rooms served as small banquet rooms—some had benches along the walls—where family and friends of the deceased gathered regularly to "feast with the dead." It would be as though Jody and I decided to host our fiftieth anniversary party at a cemetery where most of our family members and friends were buried and placed our drinks on top of the headstones.

Some cultures (including my own traditional Chinese culture) still celebrate meals with the departed; but for most moderns, placing oneself in such intimate proximity to death seems macabre and aversive to modern sensibilities. I confess I had the same initial reaction when touring the catacombs. But that says as much about our culture's avoidance instincts as it does about the early Christians' intentionality in training themselves—and their children—to be acquainted with scenes of death.

Why stock their minds with such images? The Christian inscriptions and artwork decorating these rooms explain the purpose. They are filled with words and images depicting the theme of the resurrection. The images include paintings like the one in the Catacombs of Praetextatus of a lush olive harvest (the crop Romans saw in their fields, like the crops of wheat Jesus saw in his area).[5] Even as a modern, I experienced those resurrection images in an intensified spiritual light precisely because they were juxtaposed next to stark images of death.

As I toured the catacombs, I imagined myself as a young boy in the early church. Every weekend, I would be filling my mind with a rich panoply of images of death and resurrection. I would be sitting next to the wrapped bones of, say, a beloved grandmother whom I missed. I would simultaneously be sharing a meal with other living relatives in a way that anticipated a future reunion in which all of us in the room—whether currently dead or alive—would feast together again. I would have joined everyone in ending the dinner party by singing one of the many early church hymns about the resurrection.

How different would I be if, instead of my viewing of Bugs Bunny cartoons, I had this kind of multisensory experience regularly filling my imagination? Neither death nor eternal life would feel foreign or fuzzy. If asked about eternal life, I'd be able to say, "It's kind of like . . . our Sunday meals in the catacombs." All in all, I believe I would have grown up to be far less anxious.

Practically speaking, we can take personal steps to nurture a healthier familiarity with death. We can make thoughtful choices about our end-of-life medical care that prioritizes meaningful time with family and resists the medicalization of death practices that may extend life a few drops longer at great spiritual cost. Several years ago, I enlisted as a hospice volunteer, making house calls to dying people. The experience filled my mind with images that the Holy Spirit continues to draw on when I imagine what resurrection will be like.

As with our need for better "harvest festivals," however, I believe the greatest responsibility lies with institutional leaders who are called to shape the Christian imagination, especially around our collective experience of death. This especially means pastors must be willing to depart from the fuzzy and hazy language of "souls at rest" and "eternal homes" that is more descriptive of a Platonized distortion of Christianity than it is of the biblical hope of resurrection. The words uttered at funerals and memorial services are like those spoken at wedding ceremonies and banquet toasts: they are the rare and precious opportunities for Christians to define the meaning of life's most major moments—moments of joyous gain and grievous loss.

Similarly, I invite Christian musicians, artists, filmmakers, and other creatives to take inspiration from the early church in the catacombs. Create this era's version of those multisensory experiences that reshape our spiritual imagination. Weave new creative throughlines that connect loss with restoration, death with resurrection, past with future, and earth with heaven.

Such a reformation of the Christian imagination is sorely needed by anyone in any life stage, regardless of whether they are facing a major loss. But these truths are only truly confirmed when tested. Trials reveal whether they are abstractions scribbled on a page or trusted promises that we hold—and that hold us.

Let's turn next to a consideration of how we can face ordinary trials as opportunities to nurture our holding capacity.

CHAPTER 14

From Avoiding to Holding

Today was an ordinary day for me, perhaps even a good day. In the morning, I landed a new client, which put my consulting firm well ahead of annual revenue targets. Afterward, I collaborated remotely with my editor, who lives thousands of miles away, to complete a previous chapter of this book. When I felt a twinge of hunger in the middle of the day, I turned to a well-stocked refrigerator (and made a delicious bowl of ramen). In the afternoon, when I sensed a slight chill in the air from today's unusually cold Bay Area weather, I put on a comfy sweater and turned up the heat a few well-calibrated degrees. All told, I lived today with more financial security, productivity, provision, and comfort than what billions of individuals over the span of human history have ever enjoyed—or could even have imagined.

After work, I also helped one of my daughters with her college application process. "What if no one accepts me? What will I do?" She bounced her knee incessantly as we reviewed her essay

(I fear my proclivity to anxiety got genetically passed to her in the form of JiggleKnee).

My wife came home from a company event. She made herself a drink, and I could tell she wanted to process what happened. "I feel like I didn't do enough to draw in these new people who came." She jiggled the ice in her glass. "I hope they didn't feel I was being too cliquish."

I knew I was supposed to listen and ask more questions, but the doorbell rang. It was one of my best friends, with whom I had planned a walk.

"My dad's dementia," he said with a sigh as we rounded the corner near the park. "It's getting worse."

An ordinary day, even a good one, is still vulnerable to loss and anxiety. If we manage to live twenty-four hours insulated from a loss of our own, we still experience this reality through others close to us. For those of who are secure today, the ubiquity of loss should remind us we are bound to join the ranks of the anxious on some other day. Flip the calendar, and I'll experience my own version of institutional rejection or social insecurity or physical decline.

The previous chapters explored how to face the anxiety surrounding major loss. The key to facing major loss is holding on to Jesus' promise of resurrection: in the end, we will get back what we lose in death. This chapter explores how to face the anxiety of more minor losses, the kind we encounter on ordinary days.

The Christian response to these two types of anxieties share a deep connection. The everyday losses we regularly encounter prepare us for the major loss we will inevitably suffer. This chapter shares a key growth step: moving from *avoidance* to *holding*. As we replace our avoidance habits with holding practices, we nurture our capacity to deal with loss of all kinds.

A Brief Review . . . and a New Formula

Before we present these holding practices, let's do a quick review of how this Jesus-centered "holding capacity" represents a radical new opportunity in our experience of anxiety. Permeating this book are various insights about how loss and anxiety are related. In previous chapters, I relied on both metaphors and math formulas to condense complex relationships into a graspable form, so I'm going to keep rolling them out. By the way, I am personally much more on #TeamMetaphor. I still have nightmares of being in high school math class and being utterly unprepared for a test I didn't know about. If math formulas confuse you, feel free to skip over those parts below.

The grain metaphor of Jesus (from John 12:23–38) was his elegant way to teach that every human being is subject to death and burial, the Loss of all losses. Mathematically, I represented the implication of this truth in the Anxiety Formula: **Anxiety = Loss × Avoidance**. Because loss is inevitable, anxiety is inevitable.

Therefore, our attempts to avoid loss will backfire. Metaphorically, if we seek to "love" our life, we will "lose" it. Mathematically, if we ramp up our Avoidance quotient—via our particular *away* or *around* habits—we multiply the impact of Loss and generate more Anxiety. This is why we ought to lower our addiction to avoidance habits.

As helpful as lowering avoidance is for lowering anxiety, Jesus offers an even more impactful opportunity. In his death and resurrection, Jesus introduced a radical new possibility: the capacity to *get back what we lose*. He achieved this capacity in his own death and resurrection, where he went *through* the Loss of all losses and came out the other side with what he lost—and more! Jesus is our throughline for a similar path. As we hold on to him and his ways, we, too, will get back what we lose—and more! This is the dramatic promise conveyed in his grain metaphor: what is buried in the earth and lost is ultimately restored in the abundant harvest of the final resurrection.

Resurrection fundamentally changes the relationship between Anxiety and Loss. While any person, whether or not they have faith in Jesus' resurrection powers, can benefit by refraining from avoidance, Jesus followers are given the additional opportunity to reduce the power of Loss itself. The more we hold on to the resurrection promise, the more the fear of Loss loses its hold over us.

Resurrection fundamentally changes the relationship between anxiety and loss.

Now let's use a metaphor. A farmer in Jesus' day would naturally be anxious in the long wait before the harvest because he had "buried" resources and energy into this field. He could lose all of it. Suppose he received a rock-solid prediction that the coming harvest would be abundant. He would naturally experience far less anxiety in the interim, but only if he believed this news.

We have good news too, if you can believe it: the historical resurrection of Jesus, along with his promise that we will follow in his footsteps. Jesus was referring to you when, after he showed his own resurrected body to the distraught Thomas, he predicted, "Blessed are those who have not seen and yet have believed" (John 20:29). If you can faithfully hold on to the news of the resurrection, you will experience decreased anxiety and many other blessings.

Okay, now let's convey this radical new possibility with a new mathematical formula.

The old formula looks like this:

$$\text{Anxiety} = \text{Loss} \times \text{Avoidance}$$

This formula doesn't do justice to the resurrection news because it doesn't convey a way to reduce Loss itself. It only tells us to refrain from Avoidance so we don't make things worse.

The post-resurrection Anxiety Formula looks like this:

Anxiety = Loss ÷ Holding

Comparing the two formulas shows why it is so important to shift from avoidance habits to holding practices. The relationship between Anxiety and Loss changes dramatically when Avoiding is replaced with Holding. Avoidance moves multiply Loss; Holding moves divide it. The more we hold on to the core promise of the resurrection—we will *get back what we lose*—the more we directly reduce the power of Loss.

That's why I spent the last chapters clarifying the various misconceptions of eternity. To cancel the power of Loss, the nature of the restoration we hold must match the nature of the Loss we fear. This is why it is necessary to understand that the resurrection is bodily in nature just like our losses are. The mistaken Christian conception of disembodied souls floating in heaven is like envisioning a final harvest of orchids emerging from a buried grain of wheat. Nonsensical and incoherent, that picture doesn't help those anxious about losing the wheat they need to feed their bodies.[1]

At the risk of outstripping my limited math chops, let me offer one more insight from this postresurrection Anxiety Formula. Strictly speaking, reducing the Anxiety quotient to zero is impossible.[2] Increasing the Holding quotient in the denominator to a large amount significantly reduces the impact of Loss but never eliminates it. Loss will still generate some amount of anxiety. Some fraction will remain. Stated more plainly, even a fully accurate picture of resurrection will leave some remainder of Anxiety.

Indeed, we see this when we revisit the John 12 narrative where Jesus uses the grain metaphor. If anyone could have secured a lock hold on the resurrection promise, it would be Jesus, especially at the precise moment he is teaching his disciples about it. Yet he reveals in verses 27–28 the profound struggle taking place within him:

> "Now my heart is troubled," Jesus went on. "What am I going to say? 'Father, save me from this moment?' No! It was because of this that I came to this moment. Father, glorify your name!"
>
> "I have glorified it," came a voice from heaven, "and I will glorify it again." (John 12:27–28 NTE)

"Now my heart is troubled." As we've discussed, the "heart" was the Hebrew locale for one's deepest mental state. Jesus' admission reveals he did not face loss with absolute calm and confidence, devoid of any worry. Here we have decisive evidence that anxiety is not a sin, but the natural human response to impending loss. As he heads to the cross—where he will represent all human loss—Jesus himself experiences anxiety.

Jesus also reveals how he moves from *avoiding* to *holding*. Interestingly, he considers avoidance first: "What am I going to say? 'Father, save me from this moment?'" The appeal of avoiding loss is real and natural. But Jesus then narrates his internal shift from avoidance to holding. He considers the path of avoiding loss, but he ultimately resists and declares, "No!" He deliberately takes hold of his Father's promise to resurrect his Son (the one who bears his name) to a glorified state: "Father, glorify your name!"

John condenses this shift from *avoiding* to *holding* so quickly it can seem automatic, effortless, and practically unrelatable to the rest of us. Such a reading ignores how this entire scene is colored by Jesus' opening lament that his "heart is troubled."

The process of getting to *holding* was far from effortless. Jesus experienced a mental struggle.

This should give us both confidence and caution. We should take confidence in how much Jesus accepts our anxious selves. He does not merely tolerate us in our anxiety. He empathizes. He has been there. He knows firsthand what it is like, how hard it is. Because he embraced human anxiety, we can trust he fully embraces us in our anxiety.

Simultaneously, we should take caution from his example. Shifting from avoidance to holding was challenging. He had to work to hold on to the resurrection promise, which indicates he must have had to nurture this holding capacity over time. At the point of his most major loss, he summoned a lifetime of practice.

This must also be true for us.

When a day of major loss arrives, we can't expect to snap our fingers and suddenly adopt a new mental formula we have not already embedded in ourselves. Our own shift from avoiding to holding cannot be attempted for the first time only when the doctor shares the biopsy results. We wouldn't expect to jump out of bed on race day and run a marathon without training. Or, let's switch back to our agricultural metaphor. What would we think about the farmer who proclaims his faith in the coming harvest without daily watering, weeding, and tending his field?

Ordinary days matter. The everyday losses in our ordinary days are opportunities for training and tending.

Everyday losses in our ordinary days are opportunities for training.

Holding Practices in Gethsemane

Whereas the gospel of John dramatizes Jesus' pivotal encounter with loss and anxiety in the chapter 12 "grain of wheat" passage, the other three gospels do so in the Gethsemane scene (which John omits). As with John 12, the Gethsemane scene takes place right before the chain of events that inexorably lead to the cross, and thus dramatizes a key spiritual test: will Jesus be willing to go down the road *through* loss or will he insist on avoiding loss?

Let's enter the scene as rendered in Mark 14:32–42 (NRSVue):

> They went to a place called Gethsemane, and he said to his disciples, "Sit here while I pray." He took with him Peter and James and John and began to be distressed and agitated. And he said to them, "My soul is deeply grieved, even to death; remain here, and keep awake." And going a little farther, he threw himself on the ground and prayed that, if it were possible, the hour might pass from him. He said, "Abba, Father, for you all things are possible; remove this cup from me, yet not what I want but what you want." He came and found them sleeping, and he said to Peter, "Simon, are you asleep? Could you not keep awake one hour? Keep awake and pray that you may not come into the time of trial; the spirit indeed is willing, but the flesh is weak." And again he went away and prayed, saying the same words. And once more he came and found them sleeping, for their eyes were very heavy, and they did not know what to say to him. He came a third time and said to them, "Are you still sleeping and taking your rest? Enough! The hour has come; the Son of Man is betrayed into the hands of sinners. Get up, let us be going. Look, my betrayer is at hand."

The story is clear: Jesus felt anxiety. Just like us. He contemplates the massive loss looming before him and feels the way most of us would: He "began to be distressed and agitated" (Mark

14:33). Jesus' instinctive response here is also just like ours: he considers avoidance: He "prayed that, if it were possible, the hour might pass from him" (v. 35). However, in the next verse (v. 36), Jesus narrates his internal shift from avoidance to holding. The request to "remove this cup from me" transitions to his submission to the Father's promise and plans—"yet not what I want but what you want." Lest we imagine this was an effortless move, note the extreme physical exertion involved in this shift: "And going a little farther, he threw himself on the ground" (v. 35). The physical effort underscores the spiritual effort required in moving from avoidance to holding.

Certain elements of this effort are reserved for Jesus alone. Only Jesus can take on the full weight of universal human loss on the cross. This specific "trial" is meant only for him, and this is why he tells his disciples to "pray that you may not come into the time of trial" (Mark 14:38). He does not want his disciples to take on his unique role of Messiah. As we see when one of them later tries to defend Jesus with armed resistance (v. 47), they will surely get things wrong if they try. Moreover, Jesus needs them to make it through this evening alive so they can tell others he has introduced a radical new possibility into human history through his unique death and resurrection.

However, we are meant to emulate other elements of Jesus' response. While Jesus does not want the disciples to end up in the specific "trial" of the impending crucifixion, he wants them to witness *how* he made it through his ordeal. Jesus wants them to stay awake and share the process of moving from avoidance to holding. He wants them to grasp the holding practices he is adopting because they will need to incorporate these regular actions into their lives going forward.

We should pay attention to these three holding practices practiced by Jesus in Gethsemane:

1. Prayer
2. Grieving
3. Community

Every one of these practices was honed over time by Jesus. The rest of this chapter will explore the first one—Jesus' practice of prayer, and the next chapter will examine grieving and community.

Holding Practice #1: Prayer

> They went to a place called Gethsemane, and he said to his disciples, "Sit here *while I pray.*" . . . And going a little farther, he threw himself on the ground *and prayed* that, if it were possible, the hour might pass from him. He said, "Abba, Father, for you all things are possible; remove this cup from me, yet not what I want but what you want." . . . Keep awake *and pray* that you may not come into the time of trial; the spirit indeed is willing, but the flesh is weak." And again he went away *and prayed,* saying the same words. (Mark 14:32, 35–36, 38–39 NRSVue, emphasis added)

In Gethsemane, Jesus explicitly signals the importance of prayer to his disciples: "Sit here while I pray" (Mark 14:32). Prayer is how Jesus held on through the anxious ordeal, and he returns to this activity repeatedly. He invites his three closest friends to come close enough to overhear his intimate exchange with the Father. Prayer is the aspect of the trial he wants to share as he implores the sleepy Peter to "keep awake and pray" (v. 38).

Jesus practiced two types of prayer in the garden—the prayer of *avoidance* and the prayer of *submission.* As mentioned, his words to the Father in Mark 14:36 succinctly express both types:

"Remove this cup from me" is his request to avoid loss; "yet not what I want but what you want" is his submission to the Father's promise and plans for resurrection. His key holding move is the shift from the prayer of avoidance to the prayer of submission.

We can think of the prayer of avoidance as the plea, "O God, don't let me fall!" It's the prayer of someone who wants to avoid loss. We can think of the prayer of submission as abandoning an insistence on avoiding loss. This latter prayer is the spiritual equivalent of the "trust fall" exercise, where we give way to losing our balance, trusting that someone else will ultimately hold us even as we fall.

The prayer of submission is the practice of entrusting ourselves to the Father *regardless of whether he helps us avoid loss in the short term.* I first encountered this practice in a wonderful little book written in the eighteenth century by French priest Jean-Pierre de Caussade titled *Abandonment to Divine Providence.*[3] The book explores how the ordinary events of our lives present opportunities to practice the shift from avoidance to submission.

The author provides practical examples from eighteenth-century daily life, but the idea can be readily translated to our modern context. Take my current anxiety as a parent of a high school senior who is applying to college. This is an annual anxiety affecting millions of "ordinary" parents. My instinctive move during this season has been to utter prayers of *avoidance.* These prayers are all variations on the basic plea, "O God, please let her get into X school."

For many young adults, the college admissions process is the first time they expose themselves to scrutiny from the wider world and face the prospect of personal rejection. While this experience is not as troubling as biopsy results, it can be a bitter taste of loss, disappointment, and uncertainty. Because I do not want my daughter to drink from that cup, I pray, "O God, please let her get into X school."

Lately, I've been experimenting with prayers of submission. They sound different. At the most basic level, I pray to the Father, "Yet not what I—or my daughter—want, but what you want." I also pray to be reminded that my fatherhood is meant to reflect the reality that she has an ultimate Father who holds her more capably and securely than I ever could. I pray this entire experience—including potential rejection—will draw my daughter into greater trust of her true Father. In prayer, I imagine placing her future in the Father's hand for him to hold. I even imagine her getting rejected from every school and holding that feeling before the Father. To my surprise, it is more tolerable than I thought.

As I've switched from prayers of avoidance to prayers of submission, I can confirm the key prediction arising from a comparison of the two types of Anxiety Formulas. I experience much less anxiety with prayers of submission. The power of feared loss is progressively canceled and divided. And more importantly for the long run, my capacity to hold on through loss is growing.

Prayers for avoiding loss are not inherently bad. Jesus expressed a desire to avoid drinking from the cup of loss. In fact, we ought to ask God to help us avoid losses. I often pray, "O God, don't let me fall!" But if we remain only in that desire, if we insist that an avoidance of loss is the only acceptable outcome, we will be stuck in a limited Anxiety Formula and limit our own long-term spiritual growth.

Jesus struck the right balance between these two types of prayers. In the middle of his ministry, the disciples noticed that Jesus routinely prayed. They asked him to teach them how to pray (Luke 11:1). Jesus gives them the model of prayer we now call the "Lord's Prayer." In it, we are given space to express our desire to avoid loss. Given that wheat was the primary metaphor and actual substance of provision and security in that culture, the line "give us our daily bread" is a prayer to avoid loss. But this line is subsumed under the overarching mentality established in the opening request: "Your kingdom come, your will be done"—a paradigmatic prayer of submission. When Jesus prays in Gethsemane, "Yet not what I want but what you want," he is repeating the essence of what he had already been praying daily and always seeks to replicate in his followers.

We can even trace this move back further to Jesus' time in the wilderness. The wilderness and Gethsemane are meant as bookends. One is a trial inaugurating his public ministry, while the other is a trial bringing it to a close. The locations of these two events are also symbolically paired. The wilderness is the place of exile (loss), while the garden evokes Eden and the tree of eternal life (resurrection). In the wilderness, Jesus prepares for Satan's temptation by undergoing a sustained fasting, which was inextricably tied to sustained prayer in the Jewish tradition. In the garden, he prays with a similarly full engagement of bodily—throwing himself to the ground—and spiritual effort.

Most significantly, both scenes show Jesus wrestling with the temptation to avoid loss. In Gethsemane, Jesus contemplates an option that had first been presented to him by Satan in the wilderness. Luke 4:1–13 shows that every one of Satan's temptations appeal to the natural desire to avoid loss—avoiding the loss of provision by turning stones into bread; avoiding the loss of power by worshiping Satan; avoiding the loss of physical well-being by invoking angelic intervention.

Notice how the test in both scenes requires Jesus to strike the right balance between avoidance and submission. Satan's temptation in the wilderness—in which he appeals to legitimate desires to avoid the loss of provision, power, and physical well-being—is subtle. In the final temptation, Satan even cites a biblical passage (Psalm 91:11–12) that seemingly promises God's protection against physical loss (Luke 4:10). The desire for avoidance by itself is legitimate. But Satan seeks to ensnare Jesus into *insistence*. The spiritual danger lies in insisting on avoiding loss *as the only acceptable outcome*. In the wilderness, Jesus refuses to demand of his Father, "You must enable me to avoid loss in a manner I define." Similarly, in the garden, notice how carefully Jesus strips his request for avoiding loss from any tone of insistence, any spirit of demand: "if it were possible" (Mark 14:35).

We must nurture our capacity for prayers of submission. If we remain stuck only in prayers of avoidance, we are vulnerable to believing that avoiding loss is the only acceptable outcome. When we ask for only one thing, we are essentially insisting that it is the only acceptable thing. This insistence leaves us highly vulnerable to a range of Satan's temptations. We are vulnerable to engaging in all sorts of problematic behavior. When I'm stuck praying only, "O God, please let her get into X school," I draw closer to the mentality of those parents who committed fraud and bribery to avoid the cup of rejection for their children.[4] Spiritually, we take a step closer toward idolatry where we're supplanting God's desires with our own self-defined desires. We are also highly vulnerable to losing our faith in God when we insist that a "loving and just God" must act a certain way. God invariably refuses to comply with such demands at some point. This causes some to reject him for failing to meet their self-generated definition of "loving and just."

Perhaps some of us don't think we're dangerously demanding in this way. But the proof is in our prayers. Test your prayers against the way Jesus was tested in the wilderness and Gethsemane. Think of the last feared loss that caused you anxiety. Which type of prayer characterized your response? Was there a balance between prayers of avoidance and prayers of submission? Can you recall your prayers of submission? Or do you struggle to even conceive of what a prayer of submission would sound like in your most important context?

When we remain stuck solely—or even mostly—in prayers of avoidance, we may not fall into the most dangerous temptations of unethical behavior, idolatry, or unbelief. But we consign ourselves to more anxiety because we remain outside a far more promising Anxiety Formula.

Conversely, when we submit ourselves and our outcomes to God in prayer—"Your kingdom come, your will be done" and "yet not what I want but what you want"—we nurture our capacity to hold on through loss, a spiritual capacity that reduces anxiety.

Every single one of us must build this spiritual capacity for submission. Why? Because every single one of us is headed for death, the Loss of all losses. This is the moment when we must follow Jesus to the end, when like him, we all fall backward into the great uncertainty that awaits us all.

What do you want to be like on your deathbed? Do you want to be someone still anxiously trying to avoid the inevitable to the bitter end? Or do you want to be the one who can abandon yourself to the Father God's hold? The capacity for that final act of submission cannot be conjured up out of nowhere, with little practice and preparation. That final act will be summoned from a lifetime of practice, from a string of ordinary anxieties that invite us to choose God.[5]

> **When we practice prayers of submission, we nurture our capacity to hold on through loss.**

CHAPTER 15

Grieving and Community

In Gethsemane, Jesus experienced profound anxiety. He also demonstrated the power of responding with a new formula: Anxiety = Loss ÷ Holding. He nurtured his holding capacity with spiritual practices honed over time. In the previous chapter, we illustrated this move toward holding by examining the way Jesus practiced the prayer of submission in Gethsemane. This chapter draws on two more important practices on display in Gethsemane—grieving and community.

Holding Practice #2: Grieving

He took with him Peter and James and John and began to be distressed and agitated. And he said to them, "*My soul is deeply grieved*, even to death; remain here, and keep awake." (Mark 14:33–34 NRSVue, emphasis added)

As he did with prayer, Jesus deliberately asks his disciples to join him in grieving. His confession to his friends—"My soul is deeply grieved"—is an invitation to grieve with him.

But before we explore the intimate connection between anxiety and grieving, let's look at grieving as a practice that is both deliberate and shared. Our modern Western culture tends to conceive of grieving as a spontaneous emotional reaction occurring within an individual.

Grieving can be expressed via spontaneous emotion, of course. But traditional cultures—like the ancient Near Eastern culture of the Bible—recognize grief also as a set of intentional choices and practices. These cultures deliberately set aside multiple occasions (sometimes for weeks after a loss) for many rituals of grief. A common one is the public "ritualized wailing" often shown on news broadcasts; it especially startles Western audiences that conceive of grief primarily as an interior phenomenon. Westerners can even question the emotional authenticity of such a ritual because it is not spontaneous.

However, such grieving rituals can lead to greater emotional authenticity by creating a necessary space for accessing one's emotions. I experienced this benefit when my father died. For days after his death, I was mostly numb. In retrospect, I was too preoccupied with the myriad of logistical details that suddenly set my sisters, my mom, and me into motion. We slowed down when we finally took our seats at the funeral service, one of the only grief rituals practiced by Western culture. To borrow the words of Jesus' Gethsemane instructions in Mark 14:34, we could finally "remain here"—here and present in the moment of being "grieved, even to death." I delivered the eulogy, a practice designed to invite others to experience the loss more consciously. In the middle, I finally broke down and wept. Many in attendance joined me.

My experience also demonstrates how grieving can be most powerful when it is a shared practice. When Jesus says, "My soul is deeply grieved, even to death; remain here, and keep awake," he is inviting his friends to join him. He signals to his disciples as he approaches his Loss of all losses that this is the time and space set aside for grieving. He invites them to enter that time and space with him.

So what is the connection between grieving and anxiety? How does being "deeply grieved, even to death" serve as a helpful response to being "distressed and agitated" in the face of impending loss?

Grieving practices nurture holding capacity and break our addiction to avoidance habits. When we choose to grieve, we are setting aside time and space for the emotional experience. We need to learn to *hold* the emotional experience of loss because we are most tempted to *avoid* these feelings when we mistakenly think loss is intolerable, unbearable, or "unholdable." This multiplies our anxiety.

Recall how each of us is particularly prone to be addicted to *away* habits or *around* habits. Away habits are like pushing away a rubber ball over and over. With each move, the loss bounces back at us. Around habits are like turning a sticky ball of dough over and over, vainly searching for a way to make it disappear. With each move, the loss sticks to us more.

Grieving practices invite us to stop such avoidance. A grieving practice is akin to holding the ball in stillness and feeling its weight.

Grieving is not just reserved for the Loss of all losses. Grieving is an important way to hold all the lesser losses in our life. When we deliberately practice grieving in the face of lesser losses, we train ourselves to recognize all loss is holdable. We realize that we do not need to anxiously push it away or turn it over and

Grieving lesser losses trains us to recognize that all loss is holdable.

over. We break our addiction to our avoidance habits. We nurture our holding capacity.

When my daughters face loss, I have a strong desire to leap into action and arrange things so they can avoid the experience. I am especially tempted to reach for my *around* habit: to turn the situation over and over in search of a solution. My daughters call this character "Consultant Dad."

Consultant Dad looks responsible, practical, and logical. Sometimes he can be helpful. But other times he produces the opposite effect of what he intends. My daughters will roll their eyes and even get angry. Consultant Dad can make them anxious.

I have been trying to balance "Consultant Dad" with "Grieving Dad." Grieving Dad spends more time listening to his daughters instead of jumping into analysis mode. Grieving Dad tries to mirror back their feelings verbally by making simple acknowledgments such as, "That is *so* hard, honey," and "I'm so sorry," instead of prescribing solutions.

I have come to realize that sometimes what was driving Consultant Dad wasn't just an other-centered desire to help my daughters to avoid loss; it was also a self-centered desire to avoid my own loss. I greatly treasure the sense that everything is okay in my world. But everything is suddenly not okay in my world when my daughters are not okay. I think this is why my daughters dislike Consultant Dad. They sense something else is going on, another energy at play that is more about me than about them. Consultant Dad makes them anxious because Consultant Dad *is* anxious. When I'm anxiously trying to avoid my own loss, I'm not making room for theirs.

Grieving Dad creates a space for their loss—which means I must more fully experience my loss of *everything's okay*. We have to hold the loss together. In the process, I nurture my holding capacity for similar losses caused by other less-than-ideal happenings in my world. The shift from avoidance to holding involves an emotional exchange. Grieving Dad feels more sadness than Consultant Dad. But Grieving Dad feels—and causes—much less anxiety than Consultant Dad. This is a trade worth making.

Grieving practices can be any move that slows us to the point of stillness such that we create space to feel more fully, provide words to verbalize those feelings, and invite others into the loss. For individuals, this can include silence, meditation, journaling, or psychotherapy, to name a few examples. Practices designed for two people can include the kind of active listening and mirroring I do with my daughters. For communities, we need more practices besides the standard onetime funeral service. Practices such as the "ritualized wailing" of traditional cultures may no longer be appropriate, but I often hear of grieving exercises weaving together storytelling, art, music, drama, and physical movement. These exercises are often offered by churches, support groups, nonprofits, and other entities. Consider participating in such events.

We have to experiment and practice because grief runs against the grain of both our modern Western culture and our universal avoidance impulses. Grieving, like prayer, must be deliberately nurtured over time, especially in losses that anticipate larger losses to come.

Grieving, like prayer, must be deliberately nurtured over time. Jesus did this. His raising of Lazarus from the dead (as told in John 11) is clearly meant as a preview of his own death and resurrection. "I am the resurrection and the life," he proclaimed in this story. "The one who believes in me will live, even though they die" (11:25). Jesus intentionally structures the Lazarus story as a foretaste of what is to come—Gethsemane, Golgotha, and the empty tomb.

One of the provocative details of Jesus' behavior in the story is how he deliberately waited to arrive at least three days after

Lazarus died (John 11:6). He could have leapt into action sooner and avoided the loss entirely. This possibility was not lost on Lazarus's sister Mary. "Lord," she says, with a hint of complaint in verse 32, "if you had been here, my brother would not have died." But as this event is a practice run for Jesus' own death and resurrection, he is intent that the experience is authentic. It must be, so to speak, a full dress rehearsal before a live audience. Or think of it as combat training with live bullets. All must go through the full experience, and, notably, this experience needed to include grief. Real, actual, raw, bitter grief.

The story features cultural grief rituals, from the gathering of neighbors in community (John 11:19) to the "ritualized weeping" unlocking and creating space for genuine emotion in individuals (v. 33). Jesus grieves intensely himself, being "deeply moved in spirit and troubled" and weeping openly (vv. 33, 35). Jesus shows how intentional practice and emotional authenticity can go hand in hand.

The ordinary losses of our lives can be a similar invitation to practice grieving. This is essential. Going through loss means going through grief. Holding on through loss means creating space for grief.

Holding Practice #3: Community

He came and found them sleeping, and he said to Peter, "Simon, are you asleep? Could you not keep awake one hour? Keep awake and pray that you may not come into the time of trial; *the spirit indeed is willing, but the flesh is weak.*" (Mark 14:37–38 NRSVue, emphasis added)

In Gethsemane, Jesus' prayer and grieving are inseparable from his intense—and frustrated—desire for community. Jesus desires to share his most anxious moment with his closest friends, but they cannot even stay awake through the dreadful night. Jesus' quotable response to this failure—"the spirit indeed is willing, but the flesh is weak" (Mark 14:38)—has been applied to a wide range of human experience. But its original context is located squarely at the intersection of anxiety and community.

The spirit indeed is willing. God's will is for human beings to hold loss together. While ultimately each person must bear some irreducible element of loss alone (as Jesus ultimately did), his repeated request for the presence of friends confirms the full weight of loss is not meant for any individual to hold alone. His wish is for friends to share the weight. We were not meant to hold grief alone. "Shared joy is a double joy," a Swedish proverb reminds us. "Shared sorrow is half sorrow."

"It is not good for the man to be alone" is the first "not good" statement issued by God in the Genesis creation account (2:18). Countless studies have demonstrated that loneliness greatly contributes specifically to the "not good" of anxiety.[1] As COVID-19 ran rampant around the world, necessitating social distancing and isolation, social scientists especially found that the increased loneliness created a major risk factor for distress, depression, and anxiety.[2]

The historic rise in rates of anxiety in our society goes hand in hand with the historic rise of loneliness. This pattern can be predicted by our two Anxiety Formulas. If we cannot hold loss because we lack anyone who will share the load with us, we naturally retreat back to avoidance and the resulting higher levels of anxiety.

But the flesh is weak. One would think this would result in anxious people going out of their way to find community. Unfortunately, this desire often gets frustrated by human weakness. For many, anxiety leads to self-isolation, resulting in a vicious cycle of more loneliness, which leads to more anxiety, which leads to more self-isolation, and so on.[3]

Even if those trapped in this vicious cycle have people in their lives who may theoretically be willing to offer companionship, this self-isolation is difficult for others to overcome. The friends of someone engaging in self-isolation often get paralyzed with their own doubt. This vicious cycle blocks the necessary shift from *avoidance* to *holding*, and people may end up avoiding each other instead of holding each other.

In my six-month period of intense anxiety and depression following my breakdown as a pastor, I fell into this vicious cycle. I struggled to be with others. I was ashamed about my weakness and wanted to hide. Even when I wanted to connect, I was uncertain I could even navigate social settings. Who knew when another panic attack might rear its head? I spent so many days lying in bed by myself. That was all I felt capable of doing.

I had read the studies that showed the corrosive effect of loneliness on anxiety. I knew I had to get out of bed and out of the house sometimes (if nothing else than to avoid driving my wife crazy and further confusing our young daughters). The only destination I could plausibly imagine—a location familiar enough to navigate—was the church headquarters. I was on disability but still had my corner office. I'd sneak into the building, nod to anyone in my path, hurry to my office, and close the door behind me. The effort itself produced anxiety and forced me to lie on my office couch to try to calm myself. I was embarrassed to be seen this way by others on the church staff, so I'd turn off all the lights in my office and pull the shade on the window. When I wasn't lying in my own bed, I spent many a weekday on the office couch in the darkness, watching the clock, and trying to pass the time behind a closed door.

I don't recall anyone—and some of my dearest friends were

on the staff team—ever knocking on the door to check on me. Who would blame them? Part of me wanted someone to reach out to me, and another part was terrified at the prospect. At times, my friends may not have even known I was in the darkened and shuttered office, though I'm sure word of my behavior got around. It would have taken extraordinary effort to overcome all my barriers. My friends naturally would have interpreted my behavior as the desire to be left alone. And they would've been right. Sort of.

Furthermore, they were there to do their own work. They were understandably too busy to figure out my complicated and conflicting needs and desires. And even if they had been willing to knock on my door, what exactly were they supposed to say? *Hey, Curtis, it sure is dark in here . . . uh, but that couch sure does look comfortable . . . and um . . . boy, how about those 49ers?*

When it comes to anxiety and community, "weakness of flesh" is found on all sides. For Jesus' friends, their weakness was expressed in sleepiness; for my friends, it was expressed in the misinterpretation, busyness, and enough uncertainty about what to say or do such that it was easier to avoid the awkwardness altogether. I'm certain that if I had asked them for something specific, their spirit would have been willing. But it would have required extraordinary feats of friendship for them to get past my closed door.

What should we do about this weakness of flesh?

One of my best friends (who wasn't on the church staff and doesn't self-identify as a Christian) simply set aside every Wednesday at four o'clock to come by my house. We'd go for an hour-long afternoon walk, some of it in silence, some of it with me verbally rehearsing for the umpteenth time the worries turning around and around in my head. He occasionally tried to problem-solve but backed off quickly when I was unresponsive (which was a lot of the time). Mostly, he was just there. He held that season of anxiety with me, and I held on to those walks as a lifeline.

The walks required nothing extraordinary from either of us. They were already scheduled on a regular day. The structure of our time was already defined by a most pedestrian (literally) activity. I did not expect him to solve my problems, and he did not burden himself by trying.

The meeting point of community and anxiety must be made ordinary in similar fashion. At this intersection, we humans are flailing around in the dark, trying to connect. We are willing but weak. We are liable to miss each other. So we have to schedule, structure, and set expectations so the extraordinary is not required from any party.

It is crucial to redesign the intersection of anxiety and community in this anxious and lonely era. Which is why I recommend regular counseling for those who suffer anxiety. The practice gives the sufferer another person who can share the load—and can do so in a routine, structured, and normalized way. If you are a friend of an anxious person, consider how to proactively offer some interaction—something like the weekly walks my friend provided me. Telling an anxious person, "Please let me know if I can help in any way," is putting an impossible burden on someone who is already confused and lonely. This well-meaning offer is likely to result in a closed door. Instead, offer something you've thought of already, something specific where you knock on their door regularly. Structure the time so neither of you is expected to do anything extraordinary other than to be present with each other.

In churches and other forms of Christian community, there exists much untapped potential to heal the anxiety epidemic. There are millions of kind and compassionate people already gathering regularly in small groups, Sunday school classes, prayer groups, and other circles. The spirit is willing. If you asked all of them, "Are you willing to care for the lonely and anxious in your very midst?" the overwhelming majority would say, "Yes, of course!" But the flesh is weak. Those same people likely don't know what to do (and some can end up doing harm if they are not guided).

We as leaders cannot assume that simply because a group exists, the members are able to hold one another's anxieties. We must provide more structure and practices to make this collective holding more explicit, normal, and possible. I've created one example in a video-based small group curriculum (for more information, go to the end of the book), and a growing number of other resources are being developed.[4] I believe the empowerment of our small group communities to seize the Anxiety Opportunity is a critical pastoral task facing every Christian leader today.

From my experience, I am confident that when a group is given a structured way to process anxiety together, a beautiful new intimacy can be unlocked. When this happens, the vicious cycle becomes a virtuous cycle. The more a community can hold one another's anxieties, the closer it becomes, which further grows its collective holding capacity, which draws people further in, and so on and so forth. New doors are opened, the extraordinary is made ordinary, and we discover our best selves.

Conclusion

I s this going to be on the final exam?"
   When I teach students, I regularly hear this question asked, especially after I introduce a challenging concept. In my own days as a student, I asked this myself (if someone else hadn't already raised their hand to do so)—especially as we neared the end of the course. We all want to make sure we've learned enough.

When it comes to anxiety, what's enough?

Don't worry, I don't have a final exam. But that question probably presents itself as you near the end of the book and as you ponder some new concepts. Some of the concepts may challenge your preexisting notions—perhaps that anxiety is a sin or that your eternal destiny is as a soul floating in heaven. Maybe you're realizing that you've been conceiving of this whole Christianity thing as something of a cosmic loss avoidance scheme. Maybe the truth that God does not in fact promise that you'll avoid loss is unsettling. *How much do I have to grasp, agree with, and, most importantly, implement in my life? Do I have to remember the Anxiety Formula? How many of the holding practices do I need to master?*

People who struggle with anxiety can especially get paralyzed by this kind of questioning. Anxiety makes us feel we are not prepared for life's challenges. In my recovery from my breakdown as a pastor, even months after the acute symptoms of anxiety and depression had departed, I was still unsure about returning to some form of work. Maybe I needed to rest more, maybe more needed to be fixed, maybe I hadn't figured out fully why I had broken down, and so on. We anxious people have a hard time getting going because we are plagued by the sense that we haven't gotten our act together enough.

So, I ask, what is enough?

For guidance, let's turn again to Jesus to see the way he approached his final test. Let's pick up the Gethsemane scene in Mark 14 again:

> He came a third time and said to them, "Are you still sleeping and taking your rest? Enough! The hour has come; the Son of Man is betrayed into the hands of sinners. Get up, let us be going." (Mark 14:41–42 NRSVue)

The Gethsemane scene ends with this abrupt conclusion. At this point in the story, it is unclear what exactly has happened with Jesus' anxiety. Is he still "distressed and agitated"? One of his holding moves—community—has failed spectacularly. Wouldn't this failure suggest that perhaps more anxiety reduction is still needed? There is no verse saying something like, "And then Jesus felt a sense of unprecedented calm come over him," or "Having finally gotten his act together, Jesus proceeded to . . ."

Instead, Jesus declared, "Enough! The hour has come. . . . Get up, let us be going."

How did Jesus know it was enough? Answer: because the moment of his calling had arrived. His calling was to bear all of human loss on the cross, and the most painful loss at that point—the one that triggered a cascade of even more painful losses—was to be betrayed by one of his closest friends. Once Judas arrives in Gethsemane at the head of the mob, Jesus knows: "Enough! The hour has come."

The answer to "What is enough?" depends on one's answer to a more important question: "Enough for what?" What is our ultimate goal in all this?

The ultimate goal of Jesus wasn't anxiety reduction; it was to fulfill his calling. He sought to reduce anxiety in order to pursue that calling as unhindered as possible, but his goal was not to live an anxiety-free life. Therefore, the signal for "enough" was found not in his anxiety level but in his calling. When the time to act on his calling arrived, whatever anxiety reduction had been achieved was by definition "enough" to get moving.

We should adopt the same definition. Jesus' "Enough!" is addressed to disciples who demonstrated—without a doubt—that they do not have their act together. But Jesus still wants them to play their role in his calling. The invitation to action is for all of them and for all of us: "Let us be going." When we are to "get going" is not determined by first achieving a necessary level of anxiety reduction; it is determined by our role in Jesus' calling. The point of breaking our addiction to our *away* or *around* habits—the ways we push the ball away or turn it around and around—is to free our hands just enough to take hold of our calling.

In some moments, Jesus calls us to rest and seek restoration. The Gospels are full of such examples, and we ought to be attentive to such invitations from the Spirit. But there is a world of difference between taking our direction from the Spirit of Jesus versus taking our cues from our perceived anxiety levels. Don't ignore anxiety. I have explained how we do need to recognize the symptoms of anxiety and investigate the complex dimensions of our worries. We need to pay attention to our anxiety.

But don't give anxiety authority. Anxiety does not call the shots about what we can do and when. That authority is reserved for Jesus. Any time we catch ourselves saying, *I can't do that until I get my act together*, we ought to ask if that voice is coming from our anxiety or from the Spirit of Jesus.

Therefore, the question now is not "Have I learned enough?" It is this: "What is Jesus calling me to do now?" Even if his call is to cease from some activities in order to recover, other activities remain part of your God-given purpose. You may be a child of aging parents, a parent to needy children, a sibling or other relation to a troubled family member. You have lonely neighbors. You may be a student, an employee, or a leader in an institution that depends on you in some way. I hope you're a member of a church that needs you the way a body needs all its parts. We never know every single detail of Jesus' calling on our lives, but we always know some part of it. We know enough.

When it comes to these assignments, you are enough—wherever you are in your anxiety. Jesus will not call you beyond your capabilities. He knows you may not have your act fully together, like his groggy disciples he roused to action.

You are enough because Jesus is right there with you. He's at your side. He embraces your anxious self deeply because he has been deeply anxious himself. As you get going, you will invariably have more experiences of anxiety. If you take nothing else away from this book, remember this: those experiences are opportunities for lasting spiritual growth. As you respond to anxiety by following Jesus, you will become more like him. Becoming like Jesus is the ultimate calling for every single Christian. As the apostle Paul put it, "I want to know Christ—yes, to know the power of his resurrection and participation in his sufferings, becoming like him in his death, and so, somehow, attaining to the resurrection from the dead" (Philippians 3:10–11). In other words, we are called to go through loss in order to get back all. That was Jesus' own calling in Gethsemane, and he calls you and me to follow him, issuing the same invitation he gave to his disciples in the garden.

Jesus' final call in Gethsemane is for you too.

So get up, and let's go.

Notes

Chapter 1: A Surprising Opportunity

1. "Anxiety," American Psychological Association, www.apa.org
   /topics/anxiety, accessed September 22, 2021.
2. Marc-Antoine Crocq, "A History of Anxiety: From Hippocrates
   to DSM," *Dialogues in Clinical Neuroscience* 17, no. 3 (2015):
   319–25, www.tandfonline.com/doi/full/10.31887/DCNS
   .2015.17.3/macrocq.
3. See Nitsuh Abebe, "America's New 'Anxiety' Disorder," *New York
   Times Magazine*, April 18, 2017, www.nytimes.com/2017/04/18
   /magazine/americas-new-anxiety-disorder.html.
4. Sigmund Freud, "The Justification for Detaching from
   Neurasthenia a Particular Syndrome: The Anxiety-Neurosis
   (1894)," in *Collected Papers* (London: International Psycho-
   Analytical Press, 1924), 1:79.
5. W. H. Auden, *The Age of Anxiety: A Baroque Eclogue* (New
   York: Random House, 1947).
6. Lisa Miller, "Listening to Xanax," *New York* magazine,
   March 16, 2012, https://nymag.com/news/features/xanax-2012-3.
7. Keith Richards and Mick Jagger, "Mother's Little Helper"
   (American Single), July 2, 1966 (London Records).

8. Lil Wayne, "I Feel Like Dying," track 16 on *The Drought Is Over 2* (Carter 3 Sessions), June 7, 2007.

9. See David DiSalvo, "Whitney Houston's Death Sparks Questions about Over-Prescription of Sedatives," *Forbes*, February 13, 2012, www.forbes.com/sites/daviddisalvo/2012/02/13/whitney-houstons -death-sparks-questions-about-over-prescription-of-sedatives.

10. Jason Isbell, "Relatively Easy," track 12 on *Southeastern*, June 11, 2013.

11. Billie Eilish, *xanny*, track 3 on *When We All Fall Asleep, Where Do We Go?* March 29, 2019.

12. Quoted in Abebe, "America's New 'Anxiety' Disorder."

13. Cited in Nicole J. LeBlanc and Luana Marques, "Anxiety in College: What We Know and How to Cope," *Harvard Health*, August 27, 2019, www.health.harvard.edu/blog/anxiety-in -college-what-we-know-and-how-to-cope-2019052816729.

14. Cited in "Covid-19 Has Led to a Sharp Increase in Depression and Anxiety," *Economist*, October 11, 2021, www.economist.com /graphic-detail/2021/10/11/covid-19-has-led-to-a-sharp-increase-in -depression-and-anxiety.

15. "The Mental and Emotional Health of Pastors and Their Congregants amid Covid-19," Barna: State of the Church 2020, April 15, 2020, www.barna.com/research/mental-emotional -health-among-pastors.

16. Cited in "Anxiety Disorders: Facts and Statistics," Anxiety and Depression Association of America, https://adaa.org/understanding -anxiety/facts-statistics, accessed September 22, 2022.

17. See Maddy Savage, "Coronavirus: The Possible Long-Term Mental Health Impacts," BBC Worklife, October 28, 2020, www.bbc.com/worklife/article/20201021-coronavirus-the -possible-long-term-mental-health-impacts.

18. Tracy Dennis-Tiwary, "In Praise of Anxiety," *Wall Street Journal*, May 7, 2022, www.wsj.com/articles/in-praise-of-anxiety -11651849496; see also Tracy Dennis-Tiwary, *Future Tense: Why*

Anxiety Is Good for You (Even Though It Feels Bad) (New York: HarperWave, 2022).

19. Dan Allender, "Ending and Beginning: Worry," Allender Center, January 9, 2020, https://theallendercenter.org/2020/01/ending
-beginning-worry.

Chapter 3: The Hijack

1. Bill Hutchinson, "'All the Pieces Had to Come Together': Capt. Chesley 'Sully' Sullenberger Says on 10th Anniversary of Miraculous Hudson River Landing," ABC News, January 15, 2019, https://abcnews.go.com/GMA/News/pieces-capt-chesley-sully
-sullenberger-10th-anniversary-miraculous/story?id=60334892.

2. See David G. Pearson and Tony Craig, "The Great Outdoors? Exploring the Mental Health Benefits of Natural Environments," *Frontiers in Psychology* 5 (October 21, 2014), www.frontiersin.org
/articles/10.3389/fpsyg.2014.01178/full.

3. For other examples of the biblical tradition of the indwelling of the Spirit, see Genesis 41:38; Exodus 31:3; 35:31; Numbers 24:2; 1 Samuel 10:10; 11:6; 2 Chronicles 15:1; 24:20.

4. See Saint John of the Cross, *The Dark Night of the Soul* (London: Thomas Baker, 1907).

Chapter 4: The Shame of Anxiety

1. See Jan-Willem van Prooijen and Karen M. Douglas, "Belief in Conspiracy Theories: Basic Principles of an Emerging Research Domain," *European Journal of Social Psychology* 48, no. 7 (August 2018): 897–908, https://onlinelibrary.wiley.com
/doi/10.1002/ejsp.2530; Sameera S. Nayak et al., "Is Divisive Politics Making Americans Sick? Associations of Perceived Partisan Polarization with Physical and Mental Health Outcomes among Adults in the United States," *Social Science & Medicine* 284 (September 2021): 113976, www.sciencedirect
.com/science/article/abs/pii/S0277953621003087?via%3Dihub.

Chapter 5: The Name of Anxiety

1. For research from a secular psychological perspective aligned with these insights, see especially the work of Professor Steven Hayes and what is known as "acceptance and commitment therapy" (ACT); see Steven C. Hayes, Kirk Strosahl, and Kelly G. Wilson, *Acceptance and Commitment Therapy: The Process and Practice of Mindful Change*, 2nd ed. (New York: Guilford, 2012).

2. If you like this exercise and you live in the eastern part of the country, you could use the *W* designation for radio stations (for example, WWORK or WFOOD).

3. I am most personally familiar with the kind of conflict and judgment that happens when couples have different fight-or-flight responses to anxiety. But this happens even with couples who have the same response pattern. For instance, when both individuals are "flight" people, they often reinforce each other's avoidance of problems. Deep down, both don't like their own response to anxiety (even if they don't recognize that's what's happening). Each one can end up externalizing their self-hatred of their anxious selves by judging the other. Or, in another twist, one person might want the other to act as a rescuer of their captivity to anxiety by balancing out the response pattern; this person gets frustrated and judgmental when the other person cannot do this. Anxiety is one sneaky hijacker.

4. See Laura G. Burgess et al., "The Influence of Social Contagion within Education: A Motivational Perspective," *Mind, Brain, and Education* 12, no. 4 (December 2018): 164–74, https://onlinelibrary.wiley.com/doi/10.1111/mbe.12178.

Chapter 6: Accepting Our Anxious Self

1. Walt Whitman, "Song of Myself," in *Leaves of Grass* (final Death Bed edition; Philadelphia: David McKay, 1891–92), 29–79.

Notes

Chapter 7: Your Acceptance Move

1. Cited in Martina Svensson et al., "Physical Activity Is Associated with Lower Long-Term Incidence of Anxiety in a Population-Based, Large-Scale Study," *Frontiers in Psychiatry* 12 (2021), www.frontiersin.org/articles/10.3389/fpsyt.2021.714014/full.
2. See Annemarie Abbing et al., "The Effectiveness of Art Therapy for Anxiety in Adult Women: A Randomized Controlled Trial," *Frontiers in Psychology* 10 (May 2019): 1203, www.ncbi.nlm.nih.gov/pmc/articles/PMC6549595; Enrique Octavio Flores Gutiérrez and Victor Andrés Terán Camarena, "Music Therapy in Generalized Anxiety Disorder," *The Arts in Psychotherapy* 44 (July 2015): 19–24, www.sciencedirect.com/science/article/abs/pii/S0197455615000064.
3. See Tracy Dennis-Tiwary, *Future Tense: Why Anxiety Is Good for You (Even Though It Feels Bad)* (New York: HarperWave, 2022), 43.
4. See "Mental Health Information Statistics: Any Anxiety Disorder," National Institute of Mental Health, www.nimh.nih.gov/health/statistics/any-anxiety-disorder, accessed October 10, 2022.
5. "New Data on Gen Z—Perceptions of Pressure, Anxiety and Empowerment," Barna Research, January 28, 2021, www.barna.com/research/gen-z-success.
6. See "Studies Show Normal Children Today Report More Anxiety Than Child Psychiatric Patients in the 1950s," American Psychological Association, www.apa.org/news/press/releases/2000/12/anxiety, accessed November 16, 2022.

Chapter 8: The Anxiety Formula

1. The Hebrew word *'otseb* in the phrase "offensive way" with reference to the psalmist's "anxious thoughts" can also be variously translated as "anything you find in me that makes you sad" (TLB), "hurtful way" (NASB), "grievous way" (ESV), or "wicked way" (KJV). Eugene Peterson translates this phrase in *The Message* as "anything wrong."

2. In Einstein's original publication, the speed of light was symbolized as an uppercase *V*.

3. See David Bodanis, *E = MC2: A Biography of the World's Most Famous Equation* (New York: Bloomsbury, 2000).

4. "3 Everyday Inventions Einstein Made Possible," Thales Group, November 22, 2021, www.thalesgroup.com/en/markets/digital -identity-and-security/mobile/magazine/3-everyday-inventions -einstein-made-possible.

5. See Alan V. Horwitz and Jerome C. Wakefield, *All We Have to Fear: Psychiatry's Transformation of Natural Anxieties into Mental Disorders* (New York: Oxford University Press, 2012).

6. Joseph LeDoux, *Anxious: Using the Brain to Understand and Treat Fear and Anxiety* (New York: Viking, 2015), 110.

7. See Graham C. L. Davey, Ian Burgess, and Rachel Rashes, "Coping Strategies and Phobias: The Relationship between Fears, Phobias and Methods of Coping with Stressors," *British Journal of Clinical Psychology* 34, no. 3 (September 1995): 423–34, https://bpspsychub.onlinelibrary.wiley.com/doi/abs /10.1111/j.2044-8260.1995.tb01477.x.

8. This way in which avoidance habits are intertwined with our natural fight-or-flight system means that some level of avoidance is hardwired into human beings. This is another way Anxiety = Loss × Avoidance reflects the reality that we cannot reduce our level of anxiety to absolute zero. Like we can never reduce Loss to absolute zero, we also cannot reduce Avoidance to absolute zero. However, our Avoidance levels—unlike Loss—can be meaningfully lowered.

9. See Tom Beckers and Michelle G. Craske, "Avoidance and Decision Making in Anxiety: An Introduction to the Special Issue," *Behaviour Research and Therapy* 96 (September 2017): 1–2, www.sciencedirect.com/science/article/abs/pii /S000579671730102X?via%3Dihub.

Chapter 9: What Do You Have to Lose?

1. See Martin B. Copenhaver, *Jesus Is the Question: The 307 Questions Jesus Asked and the 3 He Answered* (Nashville: Abingdon, 2014).

Chapter 10: How We Try to Avoid Loss

1. "Posttraumatic Stress Disorder: What Is Exposure Therapy?" American Psychological Association (July 2017), www.apa.org /ptsd-guideline/patients-and-families/exposure-therapy.pdf.

Chapter 11: Getting Back What We Lose

1. Quoted in Colleen de Bellefonds, "Why Ice Baths Can Help You Bounce Back from Tough Workouts," *Men's Health*, March 11, 2019, www.menshealth.com/fitness/a26788252/ice-bath -benefits.
2. C. S. Lewis spoke about this aspect of eternity beautifully in his sermon "The Weight of Glory," preached originally in the Church of St Mary the Virgin, Oxford, on June 8, 1942 (see *The Weight of Glory* [1942; repr. Grand Rapids: Eerdmans, 1965], 8–12).
3. Wright has done more than any other Christian thinker alive today to reground Christian thinking in the true biblical hope of resurrection of the body and redemption of the world. I owe much of my approach to this chapter to him (and wouldn't be offended if you put this book down to go read Wright's *Surprised by Hope* [New York: HarperOne, 2008]).
4. Curtis Chang, *Engaging Unbelief: A Captivating Strategy from Augustine and Aquinas* (Downers Grove, IL: InterVarsity, 2001), 82–93.
5. Some theologians cite verses like 1 Thessalonians 4:13–18 to argue the interim state will be more akin to restful sleep.

Chapter 12: Throughlines to Eternity

1. Morgan Mussell, "Throughlines in Novels and Screenplays," The First Gates, March 29, 2011, https://thefirstgates.com/2011/03/29/throughlines-in-novels-and-screenplays.
2. Tosin Thompson, "Young People's Climate Anxiety Revealed in Landmark Survey," *Nature* News, September 22, 2021, www.nature.com/articles/d41586-021-02582-8.
3. See Nikita A. Nekliudov et al., "Excessive Media Consumption about COVID-19 Is Associated with Increased State Anxiety: Outcomes of a Large Online Survey in Russia, *Journal of Medical Internet Research* 22, no. 9 (September 2020), www.jmir.org/2020/9/e20955.
4. See Tom Fleischman, "Study: More Exposure to Political TV Ads Heightens Anxiety," *Cornell Chronicle*, April 12, 2021, https://news.cornell.edu/stories/2021/04/study-more-exposure-political-tv-ads-heightens-anxiety.

Chapter 13: Nurturing Our Imagination

1. *Book of Common Prayer* (New York: Seabury, 1977), 423.
2. For those called to this kind of thoughtful hospitality, I highly recommend Priya Parker's book *The Art of Gathering: How We Meet and Why It Matters* (New York: Riverhead, 2018). Parker is not (to my knowledge) a Christian, but Christians have a great deal to learn from her about how to host parties with greater spiritual depth and intentionality. Her book was a great inspiration in terms of the way Jody and I planned our anniversary party.
3. Western culture's extreme aversion of death was especially documented by social anthropologist Ernest Becker's Pulitzer Prize–winning book *The Denial of Death* (1973; repr., New York: Free Press, 1997).
4. Scholars believe this for several reasons. Persecutions of Christians in Rome were rare and sporadic, whereas the practice of Christians meeting in catacombs was consistent and even

grew during times of religious freedom. Most convincingly, the evidence shows that Christians kept digging deeper to create new rooms, even when rooms already were available in the upper layers (to use if hiding were the motivating factor). The reason Christians kept digging new meeting rooms in these deeper layers is that the more recently deceased bodies were placed in the deeper, freshly dug layers. The Christians who were creating these new rooms were seeking to remain close to the bodies of their recently departed family and friends.

5. "Olive Harvest, fresco, Catacombs of Praetextatus, Rome, Italy," photo by DeAgostini/Getty Images, January 1, 2002, www.gettyimages.com/detail/news-photo/olive-harvest-fresco -catacombs-of-praetextatus-rome-italy-news-photo/157408915. For another example of catacomb images, see "Italy-Catacomb -Domitilla-Archeology-Heritage-Culture, Rome, Italy," photo by Andreas Solaro/AFP via Getty Images, May 30, 2017, www.gettyimages.com/detail/news-photo/detail-of-the-restored -fresco-of-dei-fornai-cubicle-is-news-photo/690143590.

Chapter 14: From Avoiding to Holding

1. Here's a mathematical analogy to illustrate why it's so important to get the bodily factor of resurrection right. Early in algebra class, you are taught how "canceling" works in division formulas that have an X or Y factor. In such a formula, you have to line up the same factors to generate a lowered number. For example, to reduce "10X" to a concrete lower number, you have to "cancel" the X by dividing it by "5X"—not "5Y." The bodily factor of resurrection is like the "X" factor that cancels the bodily factor of feared loss—whereas the disembodied factor of floating souls is like a totally different "Y" factor that does not cancel the loss. I think Mrs. Stuckey, my 8th grade math teacher, would be proud of me for coming up with that one.

2. The math nerds out there will know that strictly speaking, the division function cannot reduce any amount to zero. A

calculation that has the denominator set to "0" produces an "undefined result" (not zero).

3. Jean-Pierre de Caussade, *Abandonment to Divine Providence* (1921; repr., Mineola, NY: Dover, 2008).

4. See "College Admissions Scandal: Complete Coverage of a Brazen Cheating Scheme," *New York Times*, October 8, 2021, www.nytimes.com/news-event/college-admissions-scandal.

5. The Jesuit writer Michael Casey aptly summarizes this process of preparation: "Jesus has gone before us. In the words of John 13:1, he has made the crossing from this world toward the Father and summons us to come after him. We will do this definitively when, at the hour of our death, we will have to summon up whatever resources we have in order to cast ourselves into the arms of God. We need to remember, however, that the quality of this supremely personal act is not manufactured at the last moment. It is the fruit of countless small choices made from infancy onward which have given shape to our will. To the extent that our decisions have centered on feeding self we will find it very hard to change course in that awesome hour. On the other hand, if life and providence have taught us to reach beyond self to other persons and to God, then the grace of God will empower us to follow Christ and so enter into glory" (*Toward God: The Ancient Wisdom of Western Prayer* [1989; repr., Liguori, MO: Liguori/Triumph, 1996], 2–3).

Chapter 15: Grieving and Community

1. See Louise C. Hawkley et al., "Loneliness in Everyday Life: Cardiovascular Activity, Psychosocial Context, and Health Behaviors," *Journal of Personality and Social Psychology* 85, no. 1 (July 2003): 105–20, https://psycnet.apa.org/doiLanding?doi=10.1037%2F0022-3514.85.1.105.

2. See William D. S. Killgore et al., "Loneliness: A Signature Mental Health Concern in the Era of COVID-19," *Psychiatry Research* 290 (August 2020), https://pubmed.ncbi.nlm.nih.gov

/32480121; Andrés Losada-Baltar et al., "'We Are Staying at Home': Association of Self-Perceptions of Aging, Personal and Family Resources and Loneliness with Psychological Distress during the Lock-Down Period of COVID-19," *Journals of Gerontology: Series B*. 76, no. 2 (February 2021): e10–e16, https://pubmed.ncbi.nlm.nih.gov/32282920; Yuval Palgi et al., "The Loneliness Pandemic: Loneliness and Other Concomitants of Depression, Anxiety and Their Comorbidity during the COVID-19 Outbreak," *Journal of Affective Disorders* 275, no. 3 (October 2020): 109–11, www.ncbi.nlm.nih.gov/pmc/articles /PMC7330569/; Jiwon Park et al., "Depression Symptoms Mediate Mismatch between Perceived Severity of the COVID-19 Pandemic and Preventive Motives," *PsyArXiv Preprints* (July 2020), https://psyarxiv.com/s4c79; Ivy F. Tso and Sohee Park, "Alarming Levels of Psychiatric Symptoms and the Role of Loneliness during the COVID-19 Epidemic: A Case Study of Hong Kong," *Psychiatry Research* 293 (November 2020), https://pubmed.ncbi.nlm.nih.gov/32871487.

3. See John T. Cacioppo et al., "Loneliness within a Nomological Net: An Evolutionary Perspective," *Journal of Research in Personality* 40, no. 6 (December 2006): 1054–85, www .sciencedirect.com/science/article/abs/pii/S0092656606000055.

4. See "The Anxiety Opportunity: 7 Session Series for Individuals and Small Groups," Redeeming Babel, https://redeemingbabel .org/product/the-anxiety-opportunity-course, accessed December 20, 2022.